SELF ES

CW00486714

A Step-by-step and Life-changing Guide to Recognize Your Worth

(How to Overcome Self Doubt and Grow Your Confidence)

Shantel Carter

Published by Tomas Edwards

© **Shantel Carter**

All Rights Reserved

ISBN 978-1-990268-12-0

Legal & Disclaimer

The information contained in this book is not designed to replace or take the place of any form of medicine or professional medical advice. The information in this book has been provided for educational and entertainment purposes only.

The information contained in this book has been compiled from sources deemed reliable, and it is accurate to the best of the Author's knowledge; however, the Author cannot guarantee its accuracy and validity and cannot be held liable for any errors or omissions. Changes are periodically made to this book. You must consult your doctor or get professional medical advice before using any of the suggested remedies, techniques, or information in this book.

Table of Contents

Introduction

Grit, tenacity, and perseverance are multifaceted concepts encompassing goals, challenges, and the ways of managing these. We integrate the big ideas from several related definitions in the literature to a broad, multifaceted definition of grit for the purpose of this report: "Perseverance to accomplish long-term or higher-order goals in the face of challenges and setbacks, engaging the student's psychological resources, such as their academic mindsets, effortful control, and strategies and tactics."

Grit involves working arduously toward difficulties, keeping up exertion and interest over years regardless of disappointment, difficulty, and levels in progress. The gritty individual methodologies are a long-distance race; it's a leeway of endurance. While frustration or weariness is a signal to others that the time has come to change direction and cut misfortunes, the gritty individual sticks with it.

Scholastic Tenacity

Scholastic diligence is about the attitudes that permit students:

- To look past transient worries to longer-term or higher-request objectives, and

- To withstand difficulties and mishaps to continue on toward these objectives. (Dweck et al., 2011)

Scholastic perseverance alludes to student's inclination to finish school assignments in an auspicious and comprehensive way, with the highest standards in mind, regardless of interruptions, snags, or level of challenge... To continue on scholastically necessitates that students remain concentrated on an objective in spite of hindrances (Grit or ingenuity) and forego interruptions or compulsions to organize higher interests over lower delights. (deferred satisfaction, self-control, and poise.) (Farringon et al., 2012, p. 9)

Diligence and Perseverance

We characterize perseverance as an intentional continuation of an objective without impediments, troubles, or demoralization. Just estimating to what extent somebody works at an assignment doesn't catch the quintessence of steadfastness despite proceeding to perform something that is fun or compensating, which doesn't necessitate one to suffer and conquer misfortunes. We utilize the terms diligence and perseverance conversely. (Peterson and Seligman, 2004, p. 229-230)

Grit, diligence, and perseverance are multifaceted ideas that envelop objectives, difficulties, and methods for dealing with these. We incorporate the enormous thoughts from a few related definitions in the writing to an expansive, multifaceted meaning of grit with the end goal of this report: "Steadiness to achieve long haul or higher-request objectives despite difficulties and mishaps, drawing in the student's mental assets, for example, their academic attitudes, effortful control, and methodologies and strategies."

Perseverance might be characterized as the dedication and versatility is important to accomplish an ideal outcome in the presence of difficulties or mishaps. Peterson and Seligman (2004) characterize determination as "completing what one has begun, keeping on in spite of hindrances, getting it done, accomplishing conclusion, remaining focused, getting it off one's work area and out the entryway." (p. 202) Diligence is related intimately with grit, which is "the constancy and energy for long haul objectives." (Duckworth, Peterson, Matthews, and Kelly, 2007)

Perseverant people ordinarily feel fit for accomplishment and are liable for the results of their endeavors after some time. You complete what you start in spite of obstructions. You never surrender.

The idea of determination can frequently be found in one's dynamic interest in conquering deterrents.

Steadiness is an exceptional human trademark that distinguishes a person's capacity to invest significant stretches of energy dedicated to a solitary objective or set of objectives. Individuals who endure can set objectives for themselves and afterward take dynamic, determined strides toward those objectives. Individuals showing elevated levels of steadiness can deal with misfortunes that pop out in the quest for objectives.

For what reason does it matter?

For people, persistence can be associated with a person's capacity to be fruitful for an amazing duration. Individuals who endure through mishaps regularly receive the rewards of the achievement picked up by declining to surrender. Once in a while, this accompanies the additional advantage of expanded information and aptitude because of the work expected to accomplish. Determination is also associated with boldness. Continuing in an assignment and coming up short can bring about exhausting self-esteem. Consequently, it takes dauntlessness to continue in an assignment despite the fear of disappointment.

On a group level, diligence can be infectious. A lone person's capacity or readiness to endure can substantially affect those working with him/her and the group. Gatherings that show significant levels of constancy can accomplish objectives they might not have been easily conceivable. The outcomes advantage the two people and the gathering. They will be bound to: appreciate the triumph; endure later on when confronting difficulties; improve their aptitudes and capacities; and have more noteworthy confidence in their ability to conquer deterrents and accomplish objectives.

Persistence is a core virtue and a basic quality for self-improvement and satisfaction. As Lord (2014) expresses, "Steadiness is vital for the ownership and exercise of a few other Academic ideals, including boldness." (p. 3503)

Students who exhibit consistency in their homework show more noteworthy expertise of substance, what's more, get preferable evaluations over students who don't endure. (Farrington et al., 2012; Morton, 2014)

Perseverance the Price for Success

Everyone blossoms with being fruitful and we regularly overlook the challenges lying in the way to progress. We set targets and need to accomplish them immediately, yet we are only human and may miss the mark on those objectives.

Disappointment towards the beginning can prompt dissatisfaction, and it breaks the self-assurance you had toward the start. You should seriously think about abandoning your fantasies since you don't feel like you can ever prevail throughout everyday life.

Everybody knows the incomparable Muhammad Ali, and when inquired whether he enjoyed his preparation he answered: "I despised each moment of training, however, I said to myself, 'Don't stop, endure now, and live the rest your life like a champ'." It doesn't make a difference what your objective is or to what extent it takes you to arrive at that objective. The odds of your prosperity rely to a great extent upon your ability to endure and drive forward.

In life we won't generally have things going our direction. Some of the time we will vacillate or come up short at finishing an errand or getting what we need. By driving forward and adhering to the assignment we will survive and be fruitful. It was Franklin Roosevelt that said, "When you arrive at the finish of your rope, tie a not and hold tight".

Wrestling the Beast

By the time you set foot on the campus of the United States Military Academy at West Point, you've earned it.

The admissions process for West Point is at least as rigorous as for the most selective universities. Top scores on the SAT or ACT and extraordinary secondary school grades are an unquestionable requirement. When you apply to Harvard, you don't have to begin your application in the eleventh grade, and you don't have to make sure about a selection from an individual from Congress, a congressperson, or the vice-president of the United States. You don't, so far as that is concerned, need to get superlative checks in a wellness 6 that incorporates running, pushups, sit-ups, and pull-ups.

Every year, in their lesser year of secondary school, in excess of 14,000 candidates start the affirmations procedure. This pool is shortlisted to only 4,000 who prevail with regards to getting the necessary assignment. Marginally the greater part of those candidates—around 2,500—meet West Point's thorough academic and physical requirements, and from that select gathering only 1,200 are conceded and enlisted. Almost all the people who come to West Point were varsity competitors; most were group skippers.

But then, one of every five cadets will drop out before graduation. What's increasingly momentous is that a generous part of dropouts leave in their absolute first summer, during a serious seven-week preparation program named, even in authentic writing, Beast Barracks or Beast for short.

Who goes through two years attempting to get into a spot and afterward drops out in the initial two months?

Of course, these are no conventional months. Brute is portrayed in the West Point handbook for new cadets as "the most truly and sincerely requesting piece of your four years at West Point...intended to assist you with making the progress from new cadet to Soldier."

The day starts at 5:00 am By 5:30, cadets are in arrangement, preparing for action, respecting the training of the United States banner. At that point follows a hard exercise—running or workout—trailed by a relentless turn of walking in arrangement, study hall guidance, weapons preparing, and sports. Lights out, to a despairing cornet melody called 'Taps', happens at 10:00 pm. Also, on the following day the normal begins once more. Goodness, and there are no ends of the week, no breaks other than suppers, and for all intents and purposes no contact with loved ones are allowed outside of West Point.

One cadet's portrayal of Beast: "You are tested in an assortment of courses in each formative region—intellectually, truly, militarily, and socially. The framework will discover your shortcomings, yet that is the point—West Point toughens you."

All in all, who endures the Beast?

It was 2004 and my second year of graduate school in neuroscience when I set about addressing that question, yet for a considerable length of time, the US Armed force has been asking something very similar. Truth be told, it was in 1955—right around fifty years before I started taking a shot at this riddle—a youthful psychologist named Jerry Kagan was drafted into the military, requested to answer to West Point, and doled out to test new cadets to distinguish who might remain and who might leave. As destiny would have it, Jerry was not just the main psychologist to contemplate dropping out at West Point; he was also the primary therapist I met in school. I wound up working a side job in his lab for a long time.

11

Jerry portrayed early endeavors to isolate the quality goods from the waste at West Point as significantly fruitless. He reviewed specifically burning through many hours of cadets cards printed with pictures and requesting that the young try-outs make up stories that fit them. This test was intended to uncover deep-seated, oblivious intentions, and the general thought was that cadets who pictured honorable deeds and bold achievements ought to be the ones who might graduate as opposed to dropping out. Like many thoughts that sound great on a basic level, this one didn't work so well. The narratives the cadets advised were vivid and enjoyable to listen to, however, they had literally nothing to do with choices the cadets made in real-life situations.

From his own experience joining the flying corps as a child, Mike had an incline to the conundrum. While the rigors of his acceptance weren't exactly as nerve-racking as those of West Point, there were outstanding resemblances between both. The most significant were difficulties that surpassed current aptitudes. Without precedent for their lives, Mike and different volunteers were being asked, on an hourly premise, to do things they couldn't yet do. Inside of about fourteen days, Mike reviews, "I was worn out, forlorn, baffled, and prepared to stop—just like the entirety of my schoolmates." Some quit, yet Mike didn't.

What struck Mike was that adapting to the situation had practically nothing to do with ability. The individuals who dropped out of preparing did from the absence of capacity. Or maybe, what made a difference, Mike stated, was a "never surrender" situation.

Around that time, it wasn't simply Mike Matthews who was conversing with me about this sort of 'keep it together' stance toward challenge. As alumni students simply started testing the mindset of success, I was talking with pioneers in business, craftsmanship, sports, news-casting, the academic community, medication, and law: Who are the individuals at the highest point of your field? How are they like? What do you think makes them extraordinary?

A portion of the attributes that developed in these meetings were very field-explicit. For example, more than one interviewee referenced a hunger for facing money related challenges: "You must have the option to settle on determined choices around many dollars and still rest around evening time." But this appeared to be totally unimportant for artists, who rather referenced a drive to the arts: "I like crafting stuff. I don't have a clue why, yet I do." Interestingly, athletes referenced an alternate sort of inspiration, one driven by the rush of triumph: "Champs love to clash with others. Champs detest losing."

These specifics are developed and share certain characteristics. They were what interested me the most. Regardless of the field, the best individuals were fortunate and gifted. I'd heard that previously, and I didn't question it.

The tale of achievement didn't end there. A significant number of people I conversed with could also relate to stories of rising stars that, incredibly, dropped out or lost interest before they could understand their latent capacity.

Evidently, it was fundamentally significant and not in any way simple to prop up after disappointment: "A few people are extraordinary when things are working out positively, yet they self-destruct when things aren't." High achievers depicted in these meetings truly stuck out: "This one person, he wasn't really the best essayist toward the start. That is to say, we used to peruse his accounts and have a chuckle that the composing was along these lines, you know, cumbersome and exaggerated. He showed signs of improvement and better yet, a year ago he won a Guggenheim." And they were continually headed to improve: "She's rarely fulfilled. You'd figure she would be, at this point, yet she's her own harshest critic." The exceptionally cultivated were paragons of steadiness.

For what reason were the high flyers so resilient in their pursuits? For most, there was no sensible desire of making up for lost time to their aspirations. In their own eyes, they were rarely satisfied. They were something far from being smug. But, undeniably, they were fulfilled with being unsatisfied. Never short of pursuing something of unrivaled interest and significance, and it was their daily obsession.

By the most recent day of Beast, seventy-one cadets had dropped out.

Grit ended up being an astoundingly dependable indicator of who endured and who didn't.

The year I began graduate school, the narrative *Spellbound* was inaugurated. The film follows three young men and five young ladies as they plan for and contend in the finals of the Scripps National Spelling Bee. To get to the finals—an adrenaline-filled three-day issue arranged every year in Washington, DC, and communicate live on ESPN, which typically concentrates its programming on high-stakes sports matchups—these children should first 'out spell' a large number of different students from many schools the nation over. This implies spelling progressively large words without a solitary mistake, round after round, first besting the various students in the contender's study hall, at that point in their evaluation, school, region, and locale. *Spellbound* made me wonder: To what degree is impeccable spelling words like schottische and cymotrichous a matter of intelligent verbal ability, and to what degree is grit having an effect on everything?

I called the Bee's official executive, a powerful lady (and a previous hero speller herself) named Paige Kimble. Kimble was as inquisitive as I was to become familiar with the mental cosmetics of victors. She consented to convey surveys to each of the 273 spellers right when they qualified for the finals, which would occur a while later. As an end-result of the regal award of a $25 gift voucher, around 66% of the spellers restored the polls to my lab. The most established respondent was fifteen years of age, the supreme age limit as indicated by rivalry rules, and the most least was only seven.

When finishing the Grit Scale, spellers detailed how much time they gave to spelling practice. They rehearsed over an hour daily on weekdays and over two hours per day. There was a great deal of variety around these midpoints: a few spellers were not really learning and some were concentrating as much as nine hours on a given Saturday!

Independently, I reached a sub-sample of spellers and managed a verbal knowledge test. As a gathering, the spellers exhibited outstanding verbal capacity. There was a genuinely wide scope of scores, with certain children scoring at the verbal wonder level and others 'normal' for their age.

When ESPN showcased the last rounds of the contest, I observed right through to the closing emotional minutes when, finally, thirteen-year-old Anurag Kashyap accurately spelled A-P-P-O-G-G-I-A-T-U-R-A (a melodic term for a sort of elegance note) to win the title.

At that point, with the last rankings close by, I dissected my information.

This is what I discovered: estimations of grit taken previously before the last contest anticipated how well spellers would perform. Set forth plainly, grittier children went further in the contest. How could they do it? They succeeded by adding up more hours and also by contending more in spelling bees.

Shouldn't something be said about ability? Verbal knowledge also anticipated getting further in the rivalry. In any case, there was no relationship at all between verbal IQ and grit. In addition, verbally gifted spellers didn't concentrate anything surpassing less capable spellers, nor did they have a more drawn out reputation of rivalry. (Angela Duckworth, Grit 2016)

Chapter 1: How To Break Bad Habits And Set Yourself Up For Success

Bad habits are very easy to develop but can be extremely hard to stop. Nevertheless, it is not mission impossible. As with achieving any goal, stopping a bad habit begins with a single step. And while that step is hard to take, it does get easier after that. Once you are willing to make the change and will work on taking the proper steps, you will see that you can break any habit. And once the bad habit is broken, it could be replaced with a healthier one.

Tips on Breaking Bad Habits

The first step in stopping any undesirable habit is preparing yourself mentally for ending it, accepting that it has to stop, and making the commitment to stop it. Being firmly committed to this will help you to overcome any habit.

The following suggestion will help you end any bad habits, and replace them with healthy ones:

The first step is to identify one bad habit you want to eliminate. It's not a good idea to tackle several bad habits at one time, that could be overwhelming and frustrating. You also must identify habits that you are willing to change, choosing one you have no desire to alter will not be successful. If you experience a setback while trying to change a bad habit, don't give up, chalk it up to experience and continue working at changing the habit.

Choosing a Substitution

An important thing to remember is that you are not eliminating a habit, what you are doing is replacing a negative habit with a positive one. Attempting to completely eliminate a habit without some form of a replacement for it can be exceedingly difficult. You may find that you can deny the habit and the impulses to engage in it for a short time, but in the end, you will wind up engaging in the habit as if nothing had ever changed.

Consider some of these situations for substituting good habits for bad ones:

1. Get in shape with Exercise. Exercise is an ideal substitution for negative and destructive habits. Exercising is especially fitting if the habit you are fighting is overeating, smoking or some other addiction. With exercise, you will not only stop yourself from engaging in the destructive acts, but you'll be focusing that energy on a positive outlet that will actually make you healthier, too.

2. Bad habits in social settings. It is true that some bad habits creep out more when we are in social situations. While being social is great and enjoyable; it is important to find social situations that you can enjoy that will not cause you to engage in the bad habit. Identify the social settings that creat the biggest temptation

and then change your routine so that you can avoid them.

3. You must take action. It is important that any solution you choose should be one that you will be able to follow, as this is the only way it will be able to work for you. You will make mistakes, and there will be times that you slide back into old actions, but it is important that you don't give up, that you continue to try and work towards your goal of changing that bad habit.

How to Fulfill Your Needs

We all have needs, and many can be fulfilled with negative habits, but they can also be fulfilled with healthy habits. You have probably developed the bad habit because it fills a need. If you can pinpoint this need, then you can pinpoint a way to fulfill that need with a healthy habit.

Of course, finding the actual need that you are trying to fill may not be the simplest task; it may take some real thought and soul searching. For example, a habit such as grinding your teeth at night can be highly destructive, but the real question is why you grind your teeth. It's true that you can sleep with a mouth guard to prevent permanent dental damage from occurring, but it is imperative that you find out the root cause if you truly want to stop.

There are negative habits we develop because we don't feel loved, or needed, or important and the bad habit forms as a way to cope with those feelings. So while delving into those feelings can be difficult and even painful, we need to do so. Otherwise, we'd continue to just put a makeshift bandage over the problem with our bad habits, and nothing is ever truly resolved and healed. One way to find the true source of your bad habits is also to talk things over with your family, friends, or even a health professional; any of these people may be able to help you pinpoint the real problem.

These tips can help you replace your bad habits with positive ones and while it takes time, a lot of patience, and continuing effort, the results will be worth every second spent on this process.

Here is another 10 great tips to break bad habits

Bad habits can be challenging to break. Bad habits are a repetitive form of behavior that becomes so enmeshed in your psyche, they quickly become instinctual and involuntary.

Each year people spend thousands of hours and dollars attempting to break free of a pattern of bad behavior, but the majority fails. Why?

Because there is no magical solution. Breaking a bad habit typically requires hard work and there are no shortcuts. To effectively change a bad habit, you need to firstly recognize that the habit exists, and then make a conscious decision to overcome it.

Pain vs. Gain

The most critical exercise in beginning the process of breaking a bad habit is looking at what is the payoff and what is the cost?

Let's look at alcohol abuse: ask yourself "what do I gain by having 5 or 6 drinks every night when I get home from work?" Of course, the answer is easy.

For you it might be, "A drink or two relaxes me," "I have time to think about the day's events," or "I can forget about the stresses of the day."

Then, you must honestly answer the question: "But what is it costing me?"

The answer may be less time with your spouse and family, a monumental hangover in the morning, alcohol may make you cranky and moody, or in a worse case scenario, you may become abusive and hostile. What is it doing to our organs and you physically that you won't realize until years later?

Once you've assessed the positive and negative impact the bad habit plays in your life, it's time to begin an action plan to break the habit.

Action Plan

1. Affirm Your Conviction

If you don't consider the price you pay for repeating the bad habit worthwhile, then it's likely you won't break the habit.

Be honest with yourself and take into account, not only how the habit impacts on your life but also how it impacts those around you.

Make a decisive choice to become a better human being by breaking the repetitive behavior.

2. Focus on the Benefits

Make a list of all the positive changes that will occur once you have broken the bad habit. Include the improved health factors, the opportunity to improve your personal relationships, or the emotional benefits.

Refer to this list every time you believe your resolve is under threat.

3. Take Action

The time to start your new behavioral pattern is NOW. The right opportunity is

NOT going to present itself in a few days or at the start of a new week.

Once you have resolved to change the bad habit, put your action plan into top gear straight away.

4. No Excuses!

Provide yourself with a safe haven in which to activate your plan for change. As an example, if you decide to give up smoking, get rid of any leftover cigarette packets, remove ashtrays, lighters, matches or anything else that reminds you of smoking.

Bad habits are often triggered by stressful situations, so work on a plan of attack to counter your lowered resistance during times of stress.

5. Plot your Progress

Take note of your daily/weekly/monthly progress in your diary or on a calendar in full view. Nothing is an inspirational as seeing how far you've come and what it would cost if you had to begin the process all over again.

6. Maintain Motivation

After the initial novelty of making a life altering change begins, boredom can set in. Continually challenge yourself to stay on target, and focus on the good things you will achieve once you've broken the back of your bad habit.

If necessary, practice a daily affirmation like "Every day in every way I am becoming a better person."

7. Set Up a Support Structure

Keeping your action plan to yourself is a great excuse if you fail. You figure: "Nobody knows about what you I'm aiming to achieve; therefore, nobody will know when I fail."

Tell your friends, colleagues and family about what you are proposing to do and enlist their support and encouragement.

They can often foresee your trigger points or notice your behavior slipping into dangerous territory. Their feedback may is not always welcome, but their support will keep you accountable.

8. Falling Off The Wagon

Failure only turns into reality when you stop trying. Don't allow one small slip up to be reason enough for failure. Accept that your action plan had a slight "bump" and then get straight back on the wagon and continue the journey.

9. Acknowledge and Reward Yourself

Daily or weekly achievements are an acknowledgment of your success. Take, the time to stop, think and give yourself a pat on the back in acknowledgment of how far you've come.

Reward yourself. Let's say you've gone an entire month without eating one junk food meal; so it's time to congratulate yourself by taking in a movie, playing a round of golf, getting a massage, or going to the park to play with the kids. Better still, go to the park and do a 20 minute brisk walk!

10. Maintain Your Focus

Bad habits can take years to develop into subconscious behaviors. So, it's unrealistic to expect that after one or two months of altering your behavioral pattern, those bad habits will be eliminated altogether.

Be aware that it's easy to re-establish old, practiced forms of behavior.

When you feel your resolve to slip, recount the journey you've been on to get to where you are now and focus on all the positive changes you've made.

Remember: bad habits may be hard to break, but new habits can transform your life.

What 'bad' habits do you have that you want to change or eliminate? Begin to transform your life today so you can be even more successful and enjoy a more balanced life.

Chapter 2: A Positive Outlook For A Positive Life

Our outlook and attitude on life all in all has a tremendous influence in how happy we are throughout everyday life and how effective we become. Somebody who ponders everything will be increasingly loose, quiet and grin more than somebody who is continually looking on the awful side, who gives pressure a chance to get to them and who always wear a scowl.

Not exclusively does how you think and feel influence you, it additionally influences everyone around you, in short our state of mind influences our day. Creating and keeping an inspirational standpoint is basic on the off chance that you wish to lead a positive and satisfying life.

There are numerous manners by which you can build up a progressively inspirational outlook and start to change how you ponder numerous circumstances that you experience in everyday living.

Changing your demeanor and not slipping over into negative reasoning will require some serious energy however in the long run the new outlook will turn out to be natural. The five primary key focuses to recollect when changing your outlook are:
1.Turn your perspective into positive reasoning and practice every day thinking emphatically.

You should set your brain on finishing each task in turn and think just about a positive result and how great you will feel when you have finished the undertaking. Never surrender to uncertainty and let yourself accept that you have taken a lot on and simply continue onward.

2.Don't let your discussions turn negative, when in a discussion it is anything but difficult to give others a chance to demoralize you, especially on the off chance that they have a negative point of view. Try not to be enticed to fall once more into your old ways, transform negative talk into positive and search for the positive qualities in all things and any circumstance.

3.Look for the positive in people around you and bring up out, along these lines you can energize an inspirational disposition surrounding you.

4.Whatever you are doing in your everyday life consistently search for the positive qualities in it, despite the fact that it may be an exhausting task which you generally loathe doing and one which leaves you feeling adversely, attempt to discover something about it that transforms it into a progressively positive circumstance.

5.Never let yourself become occupied or tricked into returning to pessimism, it sets aside effort to change the manner in which you feel and think and on the off chance that you have been down on yourself and the world for quite a while then your new outlook will require a long time to enlist and remain around.

You will discover after some time that numerous parts of your life can be changed just by changing your outlook from a negative one to a progressively positive. You will find that your confidence improves, you become progressively well known, you feel more joyful and are more sure than previously, you can handle the errands you once loathed without them causing you stress and nervousness and your connections improve. These are only a couple of the territories where you can self-improve and increase a progressively inspirational outlook and consequently lead an increasingly positive life.

Chapter 3: Discrimination Faced By Women In Work Area

When we tackled the struggle of attaining self-love and how we can deal with it in order to achieve more of it in our lives.

Accept yourself and be compassionate.

In our daily lives, we never have the control over the things around of us. For example, we cannot change the behaviors and approaches of other people towards us. We cannot change our physical appearance i.e., skin/eyes color, hair style, natural body language etc. The only thing in which we can control is our own perception of ourselves. Take all of the unpleasant events or rude behaviors you have received from the other people with a pinch of salt. This doesn't mean blind acceptance, boundaries are important, but accepting that you cannot change people or past events can go a long way towards healing.

Be thankful

After passing through your choppy past, finally you're in the present moment now. So, be thankful that you have been shown the lessons you needed to learn and if you do the necessary work on yourself then hopefully you will be rewarded for facing your own personal 'dark knight of the soul'.

Be positive and keep in mind that the whole of the day, and indeed the rest of your life, is ahead and that your best years are yet to come! Be determined and don't sweat the small stuff. Sometimes our worst nightmares can actually, in hindsight, become our greatest gifts. If you can change the way you view things, then the things you view can change.

Remember also everyone is fighting their own battles in life. Again that's not to say that you should put up with whatever they throw at you, but having that awareness that many of us are also struggling can sometimes make it easier to understand why some people behave the way they do.

Dealing with depression

Depression is the enemy of self-esteem. It is a factor which devastates your comfort zone even if good things are happening to you. So, try to become aware when depression sets in because this element will tear up your self-confidence as you start to talk negatively about yourself.

Identify the source of the depression. This act may be one of the best things that you can do to develop a higher level of self-love. Because some people don't bother to undergo this process which results in the lack of healing your wounds.

Bad things may happen to everyone in normal life. So watch your thoughts and if you feel yourself slipping away into a sea of negativity shift your energy, maybe a walk in nature or a yoga class. It's easy to slip into a depression if you lack self-esteem, being aware of this fact is the first part of protecting yourself. Be brave and do what you need to do to overcome these hurdles.

Resolve relationships or set healthy boundaries

Sometimes we have tough decisions to make. People who we love, close friends or work colleagues can constantly test our patience to the limits. Many people in this World are damaged and feel the need to damage others. Knowing whether to forgive or set healthy boundaries is key. There is a general misconception that just because someone is family or a blood relative that we constantly have to go back to the empty bowl like a dog. You have the right to walk away from ANYONE in your life who oversteps the mark.

Oftentimes we will stay for months or years longer than we should in unhealthy and toxic relationships which only end up damaging us more in the long run.

Sometimes we get so used to being treated like dirt that it becomes a vicious cycle that we seemingly cannot escape.

The good news is that you can escape, and on the path of developing self-esteem, hanging around energy vampires is not going to get you where you need to go!

There is nothing wrong with forgiveness, but only when you feel ready. Has the person apologized? Do they feel remorse? Healthy boundaries are critical on the path of self-love. It can feel scary at first but you'll eventually be glad you put them in and will probably wonder why you hadn't done it earlier in the end!

On the contrary, if you do decide to forgive a person do so wholeheartedly. There is no point in bringing up dirt from the past time and again if you already decided to forgive and move on.

As always balance is key, healthy boundaries is right up there when you're talking about a healthy self-esteem.

History

Even though people often think of confidence and self-esteem as closely related terms, there are several things that make them different. As you read these comparisons, reflect on what areas of your life you may be struggling in. Make a mental note of scenarios that seem familiar to you. We'll use these in the next chapter to help you develop self-awareness.

Self-Confidence is Situational

One of the major differences between self-confidence and self-esteem is how they present. Someone who has high self-esteem generally feels good about themselves regardless of the circumstances. If they feel positive about their role as an employee, they generally feel positive about the role they play at home and outside of the workplace. Self-confidence, by contrast, may change based on the situation. Someone may be very confident in their ability to lead or work in a team, but lack confidence when it comes to crunching numbers or playing sports. It is possible to be confident in one area of life without feeling confident in another. This makes self-confidence domain-specific, while self-esteem spans across all areas of life.

One clear-cut example of this is retired tennis professional Andre Agassi, who is considered as one of the leading tennis players of all time. It is clear that Agassi is confident in his tennis abilities, despite later claims that he hated the sport. Even though Agassi excelled in tennis, however, he lacked self-esteem and a general feeling of confidence in other areas of his life. Recently, he has shared his story about depression, anxiety, and drug abuse, making it clear that even people who are confident or successful in their chosen life path can struggle with low self-esteem.

Building Self-Confidence vs. Building Self-Esteem

Generally speaking, it is also easier to build self-confidence than self-esteem. Self-confidence can be built simply by practicing or being good at something. As people move through their lives, they have achievements and their lists of abilities and accomplishments continue to grow. Even though these achievements build a self-confidence, they do little to improve self-love. A person's self-esteem cannot be accomplished by building a repertoire of skills if those skills do not add to a person's value of themselves.

Factors that Influence Self-Esteem

Self-esteem is something that develops over time. When you are young, self-esteem is something satisfied externally. People like friends at school, siblings, parents, and other relatives you are close to play a major role in how you feel about yourself. When they give positive feedback, it helps build self-esteem. Likewise, the way they treat you influences how you feel about your impact in the world.

One of the reasons that some people struggle with self-esteem is because they were not given positive support and reinforcement that they needed to know their worthiness in the world. Children with low self-esteem only continue to struggle as teenagers. Even if they are given approval from their peers, they still might struggle with the judgment or criticism from their parents. There are also many factors that influence self-esteem once you are an adult. This includes:

- Your perception of others
- How others see you
- The way that you think about others
- Experience at work or in school
- Presence of disability or illness
- Religious or cultural traditions

Within these different factors, the ones that you have the most control over are your thoughts and your position. You'll notice that many of the strategies provided for growing your self-esteem focus on changing your thoughts and the way you see the world around you. This allows change to happen from the inside out.

Explanation of discrimination faced by women

Affirmative action is a set of policies and initiatives designed to help eliminate past and present discrimination based on race, color, sex or national origin. In modern usage, however, discrimination is usually considered unfavorable.

This Case Study shall discuss unfavorable discrimination in relation to Nigerian customary law of inheritance, particularly as it affects women generally, widows, the girl child which touches on discrimination based on sex, and as it affects illegitimate persons, which hinges on discrimination based on the circumstances of a person's birth.

Discrimination in relation to customary rules of inheritance, particularly as it affects women and illegitimate persons, is a real and live issue in various Nigerian communities today, despite the changes in the law purporting to affect, change or correct these practices.

However, discrimination is not limited to Nigeria but a global phenomenon practiced even among the civilized countries of the world, such as United

States of America, India, South African, et cetera. In the United States for instance, the discriminatory principle of separate but equal which was used against persons on the basis of race and color was prevalent for forty-six years between 1896 when it was given judicial approval by the United States Supreme Court in the case of Plessy v. Ferguson and 1954 when the same United States Supreme Court overruled itself in the case of Brown v. Board of Education. In India, long years of discrimination based on the caste system existed, whereby persons at the bottom castes known as the untouchables were discriminated against, made poor and targets of violence, oppression and exclusion. In South Africa there was also long years of discrimination introduced by Apartheid South African government as an official policy based on race and gender. These practices are now fizzling away by the policies of affirmative action introduced by the government of these respective governments to reverse these discriminatory practices.

The Nigerian equivalent of affirmative action is the federal character principle that was introduced into various sections of the 1999 constitution. Unfortunately, no aspect of this principle addressed the problem of discrimination against women, illegitimate persons and other groups.

In the more recent case of Sokwo v. Kpongbo the Nigerian Supreme Court restated this position thus:

It is a settled principle of law that customary law is a question of fact to be proved by evidence. The onus is on the party alleging the existence of a particular custom. He must call credible evidence to establish the existence. Although it is also settled that where a custom has been sufficiently decided upon by the court, judicial notice of the same can be take and court will not require further proof of the same custom.

If indeed law is an instrument of social engineering and an instrument of development, as has been echoed by scholars of jurisprudence, then the attitude of judicial institutions should be to use the instrumentally of the law to meet changing socio-economic circumstances. Happily, however, and as will be shown in this research, the provision of the 1999 constitution, recent judicial decisions, and the provision of international human rights instruments have risen up to the occasion. It will be shown in the course of this Study that the present position of the Nigerian law has outlawed these discriminatory rules of customary inheritance. What is needed at this point is not mere codification or reform of existing customary practices, as has been suggested at some quarters, but to bridge the gap now existing between the present position of the Nigerian law and the practice in the various Nigerian communities.

Chapter 4: Limiting Beliefs Reduces Self-Esteem

"Life's but a walking shadow,
a poor player that struts and
frets his hour upon the stage
and then is heard no more."
-Shakespeare

Albert Ellis, one of the most noted psychologists of the 20th Century, presented a theory that people tend to incorporate many irrational and limiting beliefs about themselves. Those beliefs become so firmly established in their minds it is as if they are cast in stone. Doing this can limit you to the point that it may sour your ability to find your own "Mr. Right," for instance. Here is a true-life example of how negative thoughts about the self can hinder or even possibly eliminate new opportunities:

Sally and the Community Project – Part One

It was Sally's job to reach out to various companies in the city where she worked in order to get their consent to temporarily hire at-risk young people who were being rehabilitated back into the mainstream community. To do that, she had to interview managers and company owners and gain their assent. She did this by promoting the fact that the youngsters were now trained in new skills, and truly wanted to work. They just needed to be given the chance. When Sally got an interview with a Personnel Manager in a manufacturing firm, she came into his office, and began with her well-rehearsed speech. Most of the time during these deliveries, interviewers generally ask a lot of questions which she could adeptly handle. However, in this case, the interviewer, Mike, just stared at her. When Sally paused, anticipating a question, Mike said nothing. He just stared. Clumsily and nervously she continued with her little presentation until she was finished.

Sally was uncomfortable because the manager kept staring at her. She unfortunately retreated to a string of irrational and self-defeating beliefs about the occurrence:

1. He thinks I'm fat.
2. He thinks I'm stupid.
3. He doesn't like me.
4. I must have been boring.
5. I'm afraid of what his reaction might be.
6. Probably I came across too strong.
7. Maybe my clothes don't look corporate enough.
8. I'm really naïve and immature and he knows that.
9. Did he notice the little pimple by my nose?
10. My presentation sounded juvenile and too "Pollyannaish."

Sally and the Community Project – Part Two

After the interview was over (and Sally was glad it was!), the manager agreed to hire some of her people for the summer. Sally was stunned. No one had ever agreed so readily before. Afterwards, Mike walked Sally back to her car. Once she had gotten in, he leaned down as said, "Would you like a cup of coffee? We could go to the Lavra Café and talk about your project some more."

Story Epilogue

Sally had imposed her negative, self-limiting beliefs upon herself in this encounter. She and Mike eventually established a relationship. After the first few dates, she asked him why he was staring at her during that nerve-wracking presentation. "I was so enthralled with you," he said, "that I couldn't stop. You were the most refreshingly beautiful woman I've met in a long time. You have a natural look, and I love it."

Sarah and Mike were married five years later.

Sarah had a choice when she first met Mike. If she had accepted all those negative, limiting beliefs about herself, she may have suspected that Mike wasn't sincere. She may have imagined that he just wanted a "one-night-stand." You can see from that true-life example how mistaken Sarah was when she initiated her process of irrational beliefs. Instead, she chose to abandon those limiting beliefs and took the risky leap forward.

Irrational thinking stems from the illogic one sees in the world today. Much of the literature focuses upon success, wealth, and fame. The average person feels that they cannot possibly measure up to those standards. Yet, society dictates that everyone should. And, if they don't, the illogic of society indicates that you are a failure. For some reason, you are expected to reach the pinnacle. If not, you are riff-raff...the dredges of societies.

Take a look at some of these socially-promoted beliefs:

1. It is a dire necessity for you to be loved by everyone.
2. You should be extremely competent, and achieve all your goals.
3. It is catastrophic if everything doesn't go your way.
4. You should get rid of *all* your negative feelings.
5. Negative occurrences in the past will traumatically affect your life.
6. It is better to avoid facing challenging or difficult situations, in case you fail to resolve them.
7. There is a perfect solution for everything.

If you don't get that job you wanted, you are a loser.

The "Magic" of advertising will plant thoughts in people that escape logic. If you commit to a special diet, you can lose 10 pounds in a week! If you get a makeover, you can change your life. If you wear high heels you can barely balance on, men will fall in love with you. If you do up your hair style like that other popular girl, you will be successful. If a co-worker is curt with you may mean that the co-worker has something else on her mind, not that the co-worker dislikes you. Your own privately-drawn perceptions may be quite wrong. Even if others were to say that you are worthless, does *not* make it so.

Using the amazing powers of your rational mind, you will recognize that truth lies in the fact that you have self-esteem and self-worth, regardless of whether or not you make errors. Everyone make errors. That's how we learn. Don't be afraid to do something even if you do it badly. Just push yourself through it and do it! For others to enjoy you, you need to manifest the fact that you enjoy being yourself. Remember that loving child you once were. She is still within you.

Chapter 5: Lack Of Confidence In Adults

Instilling confidence in adults is more difficult than in children. Children are more resilient. They can gain confidence that has not been instilled in them. Adults are a totally different project.

Many adults do not have confidence. They are afraid to try new things. They may have fears and phobias.

Lack of confidence in an adult may be represented by some of the following signs or behavioral patterns:

- Depression
- Neurosis
- Anxiety
- Eating Disorders
- Aggressive Behavior
- Antisocial Behavior
- Clumsy Behavior
- Mental Illness
- Physical Violence

- Alcoholism or Other Addictions
- Codependent Conduct.

Depression and anxiety go hand in hand. Once you get to the root of the depression, you will most likely find a lack of confidence. An individual who is afraid of something he or she doesn't know, or has no faith in him or herself or others, usually manifests this way.

There are several types of anxiety, including social anxiety. People with a lack of confidence often suffer from social anxiety, a condition that was recently discovered.

Surprisingly, D.Osmond, who was once the idol of millions of teenage girls, admitted that he suffers from social anxiety. As for D.Osmond, it might be hard to believe he lacked confidence.

The lack of confidence in Osmond apparently came when he was no longer worshipped by millions but found himself on the verge of oblivion at the age of 23.

There is a mocking joke that states that the three saddest words in English are "Ex-child star". D.Osmond had to wear that label. So did many other stars.

How many of them are in jail? Dead from drug overdose or addictions?

The fact that Hollywood no longer wants him can shatter his confidence and he will be a failure at the age of 17.

And that's what happens with ex-star kids. Many of them suffer from lack of confidence which leads to other dangerous behaviors.

Fortunately for D.Osmond, he had his faith. As a devout Mormon, Osmond was surrounded by a large family, and he is still married to his wife and they have several children. However, both he and his sister, who were once the most important idols of the '70s, suffered from mental disorders.

And it is good to suppose that they were both swept away by an avalanche of attention that suddenly withdrew. Adolescence is a difficult time anyway. Imagine being labeled a "failure" when you're supposed to be getting started in life.

Singer K.Carpenter was another icon of the '70s. Unfortunately, even though she came from a supportive family, she lacked self-confidence because of her appearance. An attractive young woman, who had the idea that she was fat and went on a diet. She began to diet a lot, which became an obsession.

K.Carpenter had an exhausting schedule. She had no control over her life. On the contrary, her life was under the care of administrators, advertising agents and travel organizers. All she could control was her weight.

This is the case with most anorexics. It's a mental disorder that affects young women. Most young women develop the disorder at a crucial time in their lives, such as when they enter high school or college.

Unfortunately for K.Carpenter , even though she had the support of her family and had everything anyone could want, including a brilliant career, anorexia took its toll. Although she sought help because of her illness, it was too late. She ended up dying of heart failure at age 32.

You will often see non-confident adults acting aggressively. Many adults who were bullied as children seem to have a resentment and end up taking out their frustrations with others. Antisocial behavior may be accompanied by aggressive behavior.

The non-confident adult does not like him or herself very much. Because he or she doesn't like himself or herself, he or she may think that others don't like him or her either. In this way, he or she may exhibit antisocial behavior right from the start "to show himself or herself that he or she is right. He or she does not have to experience the pain of rejection, even if he or she rejects him or herself first.

Clumsy behavior is often found in people who lack confidence. They are always dropping things, injuring themselves, or simply appearing reckless.

That's because they don't even have enough confidence to keep a tea set or head in the right direction. Lack of confidence will cause you to question everything you do. It always feels like you're going to make a mistake, so it will seem clumsy.

Violent behavior can be accompanied by lack of confidence and anti-social behavior. It is also accompanied by alcoholism and other addictions, many of which result from self-medication due to the fact that you are suffering from a lack of confidence.

Mark is a person who suffers from a lack of self-esteem. Although handsome and kind, Mark was bullied in high school and never really got over it. He married his high school sweetheart, who was the first girl to date him.

For Mark, it wasn't uncommon to turn to drinking when he was in high school. It made him feel more sociable and able to talk to people.

And because he grew up with an abusive father, he didn't really have many opportunities. At 17, he had already dropped out of high school and was selling drugs.

He moved out of his parents' house and away from his abusive father. But he could never get his father away from his head.

Mark married his high school sweetheart and quickly had two children.

Although he never abused the children, he started beating his wife. And his alcoholism way was a spiral out of control. It didn't take long for his wife to kick him out of the house.

After that, Mark started dating a woman named Alice. She, like Mark, had grown up in a house where abusive alcoholism ruled. She was used to men beating women because she had seen her father beat her mother frequently. Alice was also a divorcee, and the reason she divorced was because her husband beat her.

But Alice lacked confidence. She considered everyone she knew and was kind to her "boring. As a result, Alice was looking for interesting men like Mark. Both continued their downward spiral. They both lacked confidence from childhood and both were on different grounds.

Mark suffered from depression, anxiety, and alcoholism. Alice suffered from anxiety and codependence. Both of them struggled a lot and then got back together.

One night, Mark decided to hit Alice in the bar where they were. The police were called, Mark was imprisoned, and Alice was sent to a women's shelter.

Addicts are bound to reach a depth before asking for help. Both Alice and Mark reached a depth that night when Mark beat her publicly in the bar. Afterwards, Mark attended Alcoholics Anonymous. At first, he was sentenced by the court to attend, and was required to join a program. But later on, he liked the group and the support.

He also had counseling and began to reconcile with his childhood. Although his father had died long ago, he learned to forgive and to overcome it. He did it through the 12-step program and continues to try to fulfill it by being clean and sober.

Unfortunately, Alice simply went out and found another man who was drinking and beating her, just like Mark. Sometimes people help each other, and sometimes not. In many cases, being helped by court appointment can become a blessing. It was a blessing for Mark, because it may have saved his life.

Lack of confidence in adults is caused by many different reasons and manifests itself in many different ways. Someone who likes himself will know how to respect himself.

He will also know how to respect others. He is non-aggressive. He does not look for inappropriate relationships. He does not behave violently. He is not self-destructive.

While there are other causes of depression than low self-esteem, those who have low self-confidence often suffer from depression and other accompanying illnesses.

Recognizing the signs of low self-confidence, in oneself or in others whom one loves is the first step in getting help. It is never too late to regain some confidence. In the following chapters, we will explore how we can work to have more confidence in adulthood.

Chapter 6: Social Anxiety And Self Esteem

What is Self Esteem?

SELF ESTEMEE The word self-esteem is used in psychology to describe the overall sense of self-worth or personal value of an individual. In other words, how much you like and appreciate. Self-esteem is also seen as a personality trait, indicating that it is stable and lasting. Several theoreticians have written about the nature of self-esteem. The need for self-esteem plays an essential role in the hierarchy of needs of psychologist Abraham Maslow, which portrays self-esteem as one of the fundamental human motivations. Maslow suggested that people need respect from others and need respect from them. As you can imagine, there are several variables that can affect your self-esteem. Genetic influences that help shape the personality as a whole may play a role, but they are also the basis for our experiences. However, your inner thought, age, potential illnesses, impairments, or physical limitations may have an effect on your self-esteem.

Too much self-esteem, on the other hand, translates into an unpleasant sense of the law and an inability to learn from failures. It can also be a sign of clinical narcissism, in which individuals can behave in an egocentric, arrogant, and manipulative way.

Why Self Esteem is Important

Confidence in one's human value is a valuable psychological tool and is a very positive factor in life in general; it is related to success, good relations, and happiness. A lack of self-respect can lead to depression, inadequate capacity, and abusive relationships and circumstances. On the other hand, too much self-love leads to a deteriorating sense of entitlement and unable to learn from failure. It can also be a sign of pathological narcissism in which people can behave self-centered, narcissistic, and manipulative. Perhaps no other self-help subject has given rise to so many pieces of advice and theories.

Self-esteem can affect life from academic and professional achievement to relationships and mental health in many ways. Self-esteem, however, is not unchanging; achievements or failures can fuel variations in feelings of self-worth, both personal and professional. Those who are chronically displeased with other those— families, bosses, colleagues, teachers — can have a low level of respect, but the healthy person can get through misrepresentations. A growing person's experience is different, but self-esteem tends to rise and fall in predictable, systematic ways over the course of life.

Research suggests that self-esteem is constantly increasing in varying degrees until the age of 60 when it starts declining in old age. However, self-esteem is essential in living a happy life. It gives us faith in our capabilities and motivation to do so and ultimately to fulfill our lives with a positive perspective.

Signs of strong self-esteem

The confident person looks quickly and attracts attention. But there is a healthy balance between too little and too much self-esteem.

Here are some signs that an individual must know about self-Esteem

- Know the difference between trust and arrogance.
- He is not afraid of comments.
- No people please or seek approval
- He is not afraid of conflict
- It is able to set limits
- He is able to express his needs and opinions.
- It is assertive, but not aggressive.
- He is not a slave to perfection
- He is not afraid of setbacks.
- He is not afraid of failure
- It does not feel inferior to Accept Who I am

Symptoms of low self-esteem

If you exhibit any of these symptoms of low self-esteem, you may need to focus on how you examine yourself:

- Negative outlook
- Loss of trust Inability to communicate your needs.
- Excessive feelings of anxiety,
- Guilt or depression.
- Believe others are better than you
- How self-esteem affects social anxiety disorder

When you want to conquer your social anxiety, look closely at how you see yourself. Self Esteem is considered to play an essential role in social anxiety (SAD) and GAD. Self-esteem can put you at risk of social anxiety, And it can make you feel worse. Such two afflictions combine in such a way that they begin a negative cycle. If you want to overcome your social anxiety, start with a hard time

Core Beliefs and Self-Esteem

When you find that you always feel sad about yourself, you probably have fundamental beliefs about yourself, such as "I can't control my anxiety with people" and "I don't have the right skills to deal with social and successful circumstances," "Such core beliefs, help maintain anxiety and can be rooted yourself in low self-esteem. While most people experience the fleeting feeling of making mistakes, they generally recover. But the other hand will determine how you generally feel about yourself if you have low self-esteem, the way you feel in a given situation.

low self-esteem

Self-esteem is a mental state, and it can be modified. Many of us have already heard that people with low self-esteem appear to be underestimated, as they are too afraid to face new challenges and are not adequately willing to completely use their talents.

Do not try too hard to think about ways to boost your self-esteem.

"All in all, having poor self-esteem means living a life of misery,"

Experiences that will result in low self-esteem include subsequent events in childhood and later life:

- comments from parents about physical,
- Emotional or legal crime.
- ignored or be Neglect
- Unrealistic expectations or incredibly high levels of others.

Reasons for low self-esteem
Bullying (with Unsupportive Parents)
You may have had a greater chance of recovering and restoring your self-esteem after being taunted and humiliated as a kid if you have the support of a relatively secure family with sensitivity. If you were unsafe at home already and torment persisted outside your home, your daily life was filled with an unbearable sense of loss, abandonment, hopelessness, and self-repentance. It can also feel like anyone who is with you doing you a favor because you think you are so hurt. Or you may think that anyone involved in your life should be unethical, not trustworthy. Without a stable family, the consequences

of bullying can be exacerbated, and the quality of life can miserably erode.

Trauma:

The most prominent and evident causes of low self-esteem may be physical, sexual, or emotional violence. It can make it difficult to love the world, to trust yourself, or to trust others, that profoundly impacts self-esteem, to be forced into a physical and emotional position. If it could not be less of your fault, you could also feel like your fault. Obviously, there is so much happening at one time in these scenarios that you may want to check out, dissociate, leave. It could make you feel like nothing. To gain control over your circumstances, you might have been convinced that you were complicit or even guilty. You have found ways of dealing with the abuse, of handling the mess in ways you realize are toxic so that you can see yourself among a zillion of other emotions as repulsive and shameful.

YOUR INTERNAL VOICE

That can often be a self-esteem appraisal technique. If that voice embraces you in your head and reassures you, then your self-esteem may be safe. On the other hand, if you say things that are negative or that worsen, you will suffer from low self-esteem.

Research shows that social-disorder patients are more likely to be highly self-critical. Research has also shown that self-esteem among people with a phobia is lower than among those without ailments. To put it another way, stop looking for evidence that clashes with your convictions. Try to stop the voice in your mind that tells you you're just not feeling good. To silence the voice, you must first recognize that it is there.

LOW-TIME AUTOMATIC CYCLE

If you deal with a social, mental disorder, it is possible that you may have unrealistic social expectations and problems to settle on achievable objectives. For example, you will believe that everyone should prefer it and never be able to say anything. Mistaken. In potentially difficult social and performance conditions, you will probably shift your focus to fear, perceive negatively, and overestimate the negative effects of making mistakes. You'll probably repeat everything you've probably done wrong in your head over and over again, and shift your focus to fear. And you try to use those tactics which you believe have helped in the past, such as avoiding situations or using security behavior.

Improve self-esteem and reduce social anxiety

It's not a life sentence if you have low self-esteem. And if, because of your low self-esteem, you have been holding back in your life, you will start making small improvements that can boost your outlook on yourself, which can only have positive effects in terms of social fear. While a medication such as cognitive-behavioral therapy (CBT) is prescribed to reduce SAD symptoms and can also improve boost self-esteem, you can also do it yourself to increase your ability to accurately see who you are and accept:

Challenge your inner voice:

Get used to hearing yourself what you're doing. But try to recognize what you've done right when you're negative, instead of punishing yourself for what you've done wrong.

Be compassionate

Offer yourself the same care as a close friend or relative. Remember what we said earlier? You are more likely to develop healthy self-esteem if you are listened to, appreciated, loved, praised, and welcomed.

Chapter 7: Highly Sensitive Introverts 'Strengths And Struggles

Empaths have a great deal of strengths that support them in living complete, wonderful lives. When you begin to come to terms with your identity as an Empath and you integrate protection and self-care measures into your life, working in alignment with your empathic gift will become easier. This means that you can begin to enjoy the many benefits and strengths of being an Empath.

Here are some of the wonderful strengths you can look forward to developing and embodying when you awaken to your empathic abilities and begin to take control over them:

A Great Power

Empaths are extremely powerful. This is one of the reasons society puts them down so much. They are afraid of their power. As an individual who can sense things about people that they may not be willing to share, or who can deeply connect to plants and animals around them, you possess clear differences from the average person. In modern society, there are a lot of individuals who are deeply disconnected from the world around them. They struggle to tune in on basic levels, never mind as deeply as you do. You may see it as a weakness, but that is only because you have been conditioned to. In reality, you possess a great power. Once you learn to embrace it and use it to your advantage, you will be unstoppable in creating positive change in the world.

An Amazing Friend

Anyone who has an Empath as a friend should be incredibly grateful. Empaths are amazing friends. Empaths truly cherish the people they love in their life and will go to extreme lengths to help and protect them. They give great advice to their friends. When a friend has a problem or some sort of difficulty, Empaths are happy to use their beautiful gift of empathizing and putting themselves in their friend's shoes to understand the particular situation and figure out what the best possible decision is.

Ability to Detect Red Flags

Because of your ability to see what is going on beneath the surface, you have an uncanny ability to detect red flags in any person or situation. You do this by empathizing with the other person, essentially allowing you to step into their shoes. This means that you can detect the harmony between the person's words, actions and feelings. There, you can determine whether they are acting in alignment with the truth or if they are lying or being dishonest in any way. By sensing any signs of incongruence, you are able to detect possible ulterior motives.

Whether or not you choose to actually recognize and act on these is a completely different story, but your ability to detect them and become aware of them is extremely powerful. You are capable of knowing any time there is something inherently wrong about a situation, making it easy for you to avoid danger and energetic attacks if you are tuned in and capable of acting on this information. If you are not yet, do not worry. As an Empath, you are capable of tapping into this ability at any time. It is not too late for you.

Detecting Compulsive Liars

Another great ability you have with being able to tell what is truly going on under the surface of others is that you can easily detect compulsive liars. When people are lying, you know it almost instantly. Just like the red flags, you can detect the harmony between the person's words, actions and feelings. By recognizing any signs of disharmony, it can be easy for you to suspect lying. This often comes as just a "knowingness" within. This encourages you to refrain from believing them and can support you in preventing yourself from getting drawn in and trapped in their web of lies. The more you practice this, the better you will become at using this gift.

If you are a wounded healer and not able to utilize your gift efficiently, you may find yourself getting trapped into a person's web of lies. This is something important to address in the process of healing this archetype, if you have it.

Strong Creative Talents

Individuals who are gifted Empaths are known to be very strong in their creative talents. As we have already discussed, they are skilled artists, singers, poets, writers and creators in general. Empaths view the world in a poetic way that enables them to create unique art pieces that highlight their unique view on the world. Their ability to visualize something in their head and bring it into the material world with their creativity is simply amazing. The challenge for most Empaths is first eliminating all the negativity they have absorbed growing up. This negativity could be in the form of doubt, insecurity, fear of failure, and lack of confidence.

Virtually every Empath has the potential to be creative, though how they express or use the trait may vary. In other words, not every Empath will be great at the same thing, but they all will have some degree of creativity that they can use to express themselves and serve the world. This is incredibly satisfying and fulfilling for the Empath.

Excellent Problem Solvers

When an Empath has developed their empathic gift, they can be excellent problem solvers. Using their empathetic ability, they are able to analyze the wants and needs of different parties from multiple points of view. By being able to analyze a certain situation and see many different points of view, gives the Empath a great edge to be able to come up with the best possible solution that will be beneficial for both parties.

Great Entrepreneurship Abilities

Because of their intuitive abilities and their superb ability to solve problems, Empaths make great entrepreneurs. They are highly focused on delivering the best results to their clients, no matter what their line of work may be. Furthermore, they are heavily driven by a desire to have freedom and to escape from the toxic, overwhelming, and greedy environments of traditional 9 - 5 jobs.

Empath entrepreneurs are great at coming up with creative companies that reach the needs of their clients in ways that larger companies tend to overlook completely. They typically find themselves in their own companies that offer some form of healing or shifting modern society. Counselors, life and business coaches, alternative healers, artists, writers, and other career paths are extremely common for Empaths to choose. Fortunately, each of these can be done on an entrepreneurial basis. They are also excellent choices as they cater to the unique strengths and weaknesses of the Empath, allowing them to shine their brightest and serve in the way that their soul needs to shine.

If you are an Empath and you are not presently on the path of being an entrepreneur, you may find great joy and benefit in beginning this life path. With your gifts and abilities, you have the capacity to begin your life as an entrepreneur and create great success in doing so. There are many great benefits to choosing this career path. Some of these benefits include:

You are able to experience much more flexibility and freedom in your life compared to working a job

You can control your own working schedule and holidays

You do not have to deal with the draining and toxic environments of a 9-5 job

You can choose the people you want to work with or work solely online

You can work from home

You have the potential to earn much more than what a job can offer you

You can put your creative ability to good use

Become more fulfilled and happy in what you do

More travel opportunities may present themselves to you

General health and happiness will improve when you remove yourself from negative, toxic work environments

Many people believe that empathic entrepreneurship is the way of the future. As more and more people seek to lead a more socially conscious and responsible life, many are avoiding large businesses and corporations that are typically known for being irresponsible, unkind, and savage in their business dealings. These exact same people are seeking entrepreneurs running their own socially responsible businesses in a way that genuinely serves their needs on a personal level. As an Empath, you have exactly what it takes to serve in this way, meaning that you and your gifts are exactly what these people are looking for.

Strong Relation to Animals and Plants

Another great strength possessed by Empaths is their connection to animals and plants. As you know from animal Empaths and plant Empaths, these individuals have incredible talents when it comes to communicating with animals and plants. This is a breath of fresh air in a world where very little concern has been shown to the environment and those who inhabit it. Many humans in the modern world rarely consider other humans, let alone other species or life forms. As an Empath, you may have a powerful ability to relate to these life forms and protect them from the destruction of humans who experience little to no empathy in their lives.

Animals and plants are also believed to be Empathic, meaning that you may find that animals and plants respond well to you, also. You may find yourself attracting animals into your life and having an uncanny ability to help plants thrive in a way that others may struggle to do. This is because they are intuitive and can sense that you are kind. This allows them to automatically trust in you and feel safe, protected and nourished in your presence. They sense your energy, and it supports them in thriving.

Chapter 8: Leave Suggested

"If you want to be something that leaves you, it will not help you overcome sins and doubtful setbacks. Never give up. For the thorn in power and be persistent. Someday it won't be - said Mark Lamour. You let your father suggest what not it is good at all, they are by nature, there is no place, people are always afraid of being able to change the destiny of those in which they live, and all things are suggested, which is a precious blessing for their souls. Helen Keller, You also want to know who is the "life expectancy to conceive the audacity, experience, or nothingness of man." To succeed in life, you must direct your powers to find solutions to the problems facing humanity. Let Eleanor He said: "This day, I would not have been scared." The courage to do it is not to be, cannot be. Alberti V. Haller's first look, you know that I am always safe. On the shore, where it is kept, but not later ". A pleasant aspect and suggested that the beginning and end of suffering and misery of it. You can not save yourself, do not leave suggested. Admirari is not allowed Jennifer Aniston is "always wanted, and what is outside is suggested." We could not have asked for the pointer; It's about people at home with you. You are a particular condition that feels independent and free to live life.

Heidi Klum is a "well done, without waiting for others to be hungry. The early worm gives you. You are the only one who is hungry for success. So, be kind. Do not you suggest the suggested period? What? " It was recommended a great enemy and such character, that no more than there is, no inspection necessary, shapes our lives, new perspectives, which are, on the other hand, arrests, anxiety. " Fear of the difficulties that even the people you have. But don't be afraid and don't reach your goals. And if you don't meet your goals, you can't be happy, or you're saturated. Howard Walsten means that c is something awkward today." After leaving the ship, you will not solve anything; What

I want can be creative. He, who sometimes feels attracted to the current due to the condition. Live in the past if you don't see the reasons to be better. "Life will change much more than walking through dreams, which he suggested," Carl said. What do you keep suggesting? Even led by my presence, the one for which one does things just to be. And does it belong to the present, not the past? In the past, if you live in it, it may not be.

"It will take us. Fear scares us. To grow, you must overcome fear, and your father suggested that he always wanted to be," said Debasish Mridha. And as Sbastien Walsch "begins at the end of your life, they suggested." I wouldn't have it live if they were still as suggested. If you want to leave your suggestion to participate in a successful treaty with people. In the beginning, it is difficult, but in the end, it is. Then, to the extent that we cannot live your dream, ours suggested a phrase in them, "- said Peter McWilliams. Where the father lives indicated that we have no free will. His ability to think freely less human and animals. Mark Pulsifer, who wants to know ", where it is suggested, would be to stay. Give, discover yours: that of everything you can assume. " Remember that death was made. Remember the incredible goals that must be achieved. Your potential cannot be seen; if you live in it, it may not be. Massage believes Alder", always preparing you to live in an obvious step when you have suggested. " I was not forbidden to appear. Victory is happiness six steps from you. Much if you want to send to know your father suggested in life."

Bill Courtney said: "Each one of us, the door cannot be. This is when the doubt is that I do not want to leave. At all times, always remember that you are out of your suggestion; it is not recommended to enter God." It seems that no space deserves this before God. However, it is not necessary to take a step, and for one, we only suggest it. Nothing happens, so for separation and sleep. Dennis Waitley knew that when we say "a dream in the vision of creating your own future. You have to go out and feel comfortable with the current one suggests the unknown and the unknown. Virtue makes a man stroke for the unknown. Victory is given in the act. You must be strong to overcome the challenges there to the other side of the street; it is the victory. of course, attention can not help but be, and so, before leaving his advice, he suggested and Courtney, Bill wants to know, "or it is likely that he will not last the life of the depths, along with the remains could not be. " Why not those who are missing the place to do it. " When moving out of his suggested that, a strange time to be great and terrible standard "Sharma and succeed in all areas of life.

As for Dale, "plush comfort zone than the coffin. When living in a luxuriously lined coffin, do not die. And any unique force he can do to stay in the pointer. St. Rashedur Carl wants you to know that he" suggested that he is Where you can increase your means caused an error other than increasing your power if you can think about it, and grow from this area. " The person who does not have a permanent place to be. Then, take and be immediately suggested these things ", as in life, we have why it is in the energy sector, but always worries about what was suggested above, "John Maxwell said, that's not how they shouldn't be for a while, it won't be, he fears for a great enemy that opinion will be, the company can't be, it's not easy to get out, it can't be, what is that? And we go to the environment of which little or nothing is known, but the truth is that you can face all the challenges that are presented to you in your life. Manoj Arora emphasized that "it is difficult suggested at the beginning, in the middle of having an um .. What is finally at the end of drugs shows you the whole world. "

Then, according to Brian Tracy, "that the course of oneself cannot be. You cannot cultivate anything other than what we think, and the disadvantages of feeling once embarrassing when you do something new. The time has come for you to have done that with the latest state of life. I do not and need to send a hand, and something is wrong with you. The need to do something meaningful with his life, and before it is too late. Do not want to follow the prompter. He fled because he was tired of progressing. Therefore, they must think that they are associated with. Marcus Salmansohn believes that "everything in life is better for the result, often as you have suggested." Time and if they are lost, others to take a bold step today. "Get out of your land and suggested that others outside yourself wyznaczyliście confines" - Giulio observed a calf not only desirable if it does not come to an end. You have the ability to achieve what belongs to you in some, for example, and in Him are all things, as he had in mind. Each Vujicic said, "not only for the lives of those in trouble. This is life. Dream, and suggested a place where life goes on. But the area is a great fear.

" In a way, you feel uncomfortable; they can succeed. If you want to stay as suggested, they do it is not necessary - Luci I Poxlietner. Residents within reach of the proposed. Why limit the power of free choice? Cicero lost the course of fear Cicero admitted that Dan "Grande suggested a hostile force; Who does not need to go beyond the mere examination of the forms, our lives, the new perspectives, which are, on the other hand, the arrests, all the anxiety about " everything we want from a suggested. He can say that you wish to Sivaprakash Sidhu that ", And we fear the other " Fear led to life. So fear broke the feel and function of the emergence of men. So there is no fear that he was still alive. Then, according to Brian Tracy," so that I can't be You cannot grow unless you want the shameful and unpleasant feeling when you are looking for something new. Life must change, if only it will not be the same for all the saved to achieve their goals. One can remain at the pointer to continue searching for his ends. Look around. You see, the successful people of the earth? Studies have a lifestyle. You'll notice that every day for things always busies looking for new ones. I hate to kill you. I wish they suggested that he can do it.

Jack Canfield believes that " the greatest reward in life can be found outside suggested. I live with it. Fear essential and in danger, we are, if we want to give rise to life adventures and victories over them. " Through patience and perseverance able to overcome challenges and be in a perfect way. So far, they know they can't grow without problems. How bad are the challenges that? Challenges and opportunities. I don't see it as expected of him. Has it all. In the most conducive to change, and not to commit the evil Eker Harv, he suggests, "If so, the disadvantages, on the other hand, a return to the past has suggested stroking us, because you say:" I am fruitful, "and continues: that for you, you can not continue, if no challenges, too little, or nothing at all, suggested the problem. Therefore, we can not grow. Jean-Ray does not know that "something great before suggested the effect is violated " and Ray Bennett" is honest, we must also accept that the terms of fear not to lie and in our suggestion of justification. " The risk if you want to have a pristine life. During personal experiences, Sherri Shepherd confessed" the secret of who I was "to scare." And if you are afraid regardless of Go, and do it only because you are so worried that they will not make you feel much better when you and your ex are not.

"I leave suggested. The easiest way is to look fresh and ornate. Friends and great people in my high school ended up in a car wash. When you're looking for something new. A whole world opens up possibilities. As bad as you can't, in that. It won't be wrong, but the strange way, carefully, in a place where you never will - said Terry Crews. Parenting question than Godoy for us. The problem is: "It is better to know the comfort of going," Cruel Roz thinks, " and it does not contribute even more unknown the disadvantages are a new land. That loss was a sign of victory, no surprises! If it is outside our comfort, the problems, stroke, that is, grow! Why he did it; So, according to Jillian Michaels, we have to "feel uncomfortable." We have to get out of the suggested. Herbie Hancock's synthesis wasted time. He said: "Do not be afraid to expand, as indicated. Joy is coming.

Chapter 9: Trust Your Own Feelings

"What number of considerations one loses when one chooses not to be something, but to be somebody" — Coco Chanel

Self-esteem necessitates that you figure out how to tune in to and depend on feelings and not consequently react to the opinions of other individuals.

Solid self-esteem encourages you to be confident, reliable and associate with other individuals. In any case, if you do not have it, feeling skilled and serving might be uncommon. Instead, you may feel uncouth or useless frequently.

Poor self-esteem can be an issue for some. If an individual does not like herself, she cannot trust or approve her own feelings or encounters. This is going to complicate every bit of her connections and associations with others, just as adversely influencing her general psychological well-being and everyday life.

This is a particularly vital issue. Self-esteem can enormously affect aspects with annoyance, individual objectives, and connections.

When you battle with poor self-esteem, you may exasperate the danger you may involve yourself in. Different issues can be restored and remain unresolved, usually left to detonate. Poor self-esteem can result in not supporting yourself or even neglecting to appreciate your own emotions. Interacting with others requires a capacity to confide in your own point of view about others and circumstances. Because of low self-esteem, you might be not able to declare your considerations or feelings apart from through indignation.

Poor self-esteem can make it challenging to accomplish individual objectives effectively. If an individual does not imagine that she has the right to get or achieve something, by what means can she indeed be effective at it? For example, you may experience issues in making and building up kinships because of your low assessment of yourself restrains you.

Low self-esteem can likewise make you suspicious of others. You may feel that a companion needs something from you or will not care for you if they truly become acquainted with you. To keep them in your life, you may abstain from discussing issues until it grows into resentment, making you push your friends and family away.

One thing self-esteem does is empower you to set objectives and work towards accomplishing them. You may not feel deserving of things like connections, satisfaction, and achievement. Self-esteem is what gives you a feeling of value.

So regularly, we are advised to "Simply trust your gut," yet what does it mean and even more critically, how would you do it?

Gut sense, or instinct, is your prompt comprehension of something; there is no compelling reason to consider it or get another conclusion thoroughly—you simply know. Your instinct emerges as an inclination inside your body that you solitarily experienced. Since the inclination is so close to home, nobody else can say something to let you know whether you're in contact with your gut impulse or not. Only you need to decide. Because of this, believing your instinct is simply a definitive demonstration of trusting yourself.

Tuning in to your instinct helps you to maintain a strategic distance from undesirable connections and circumstances. Every day in your life, numerous individuals will have thoughts regarding what's best for you, some held with well-meaning plans and some originating from a position of misleading, unsafe, egocentric expectation. It's occasionally difficult to tell which the class which an individual falls into, however, if you set aside those external suppositions and instead tune in to the persuasion of your own instinct, it will direct you to what is really best for you.

The way toward believing your gut is not as easy as the expression suggests, mainly when certain habits and conditions pull us firmly and frequently unknowingly the other way. Fortunately, our instinct is so profoundly instinctual that regardless of whether we have been withdrawn from it for our whole lives, it is still there within us, hanging tight for us to call its insight.

Your instinct resembles your very own North Star, but numerous obstructers go about as mists reducing its light. When you are mindful of them, you will better catch yourself when you are going off course for the misguided reasons so you would then be able to find a way to realign with your instinct. These are the guilty parties:

Overthinking: Since instinct is characterized as "the capacity to comprehend something intuitively, without the requirement for cognizant thinking," overthinking is one of the most significant obstacles. Putting final thoughts into each choice and strolling through many situations and results can lead you far from your gut intuition, particularly when you are overthinking to legitimize or validate something. In these cases, your perspective is not streaming openly or naturally but is following a quite specific plan to fabricate evidence for something you have officially decided on. In different cases, the surge of potential outcomes and contemplations that overthinking creates can overpower and befuddled, leaving you in a confounding circle without clear heading. This state is alluded to as analysis paralysis. Regardless of the correct procedure, overthinking drives you to a similar spot—withdrawn from your gut nature.

"Shoulds": "Shoulds" frequently enter the picture when you are overthinking and different occasions when you are apparently engaged. For instance, if you wonder, "Will [someone else] likes me if I do this?" In these examples, you're contemplating your conduct in a focal point shaded by the standards, inclinations, and desires that another person has set as opposed to searching internally and allowing your own thoughts and enabling your own considerations and requirements to control your conduct, which would lead you to pose a different inquiry like, "How will I feel about myself if I do this?" Because "shoulds" move the

concentrate far from you, they separate you from your instinct.

Prejudices and Unconscious Bias: Even though preferences and oblivious inclinations are in one way or the other quite contrary to overthinking, they effectively affect your instinct. Rather than overthinking and over-investigation, prejudices, and unconscious bias work from snappy decisions that the cerebrum naturally makes dependent on past encounters, generalizations, and foundation rather than dependent on reason or genuine encounter. Thus, neither of these offenders enables space for you to take advantage of the experiential idea of instinct.

A friend or family members' or influential figure's needs/requirements/assessment/guidance: Often, the individual who has the best capacity to shroud or cloud your gut intuition, is a friend or family member or expert figure whose adoration or endorsement you wish to prevail upon, for instance, a parent, partner, instructor, or mentor.

When you gravely need something: When you are incredibly hungry for something, regardless of whether love, acknowledgment, kids, societal position, or something different, your powerful urge to fill that vast need can make you disregard or overlook any warnings en-route. Being laser-centered around fulfilling a need you consider deserving practically leaves little chance to recognize or pursue your instinct, mainly if that gut intuition is inconsistent with a person or something firmly lined up with this need.

Past torture/abuse in childhood: Perhaps the most overwhelming of the considerable number of guilty parties is having encountered mistreatment and violence as a kid. Why? Since youth, treatment can leave an enduring effect on an individual that can remain even in adulthood. Growing up encountering physical, sentimental/mental, or potentially sexual abuse can make kids doubt their experience and accuse themselves. Since believing your instinct is merely equivalent to understanding, taking advantage of this gut intuition can be a battle.

When you are living in a sheltered life and hurrying all over, regardless of whether physically or rationally, you miss information. Slackening encourages you had better perceive and procedure the information you get, in your psyche as well as in your body. To do such, you should rationally and physically clean up the messiness. In reality, it may look like pushing back a due date to expel direness from a choice. It could likewise mean venturing far from a circumstance to increase further precision, for example getting away before making a profession change or investing some energy away from your partner to decide whether you are right for one another.

Slackening alludes consciously making space for your instinct to involve. The slower pace helps moves your point of view and gathers up diversions so that you can see and feel what genuinely makes a difference. Check out reflection, yoga, careful breathing activities, and different practices that move your concentration from running thoughts into a deeper space of quiet and focused attention inside you.

Instinct is grounded inside the sensations within the body, so figuring out how to perceive what is happening inside your body—for example, what you are feeling—is critical to building up your instinct. While we may utilize the expressions "feelings" and "sensations" conversely to portray instinct, note the slight difference here: mainly, we're increasingly keen on seeing how your body feels in reaction to a feeling—for instance, outrage feels tight, sore, hot, and tingly—instead of basically naming a feeling like bitter, irate, or baffled, and ceasing there. An incredible method to practice is to recall the mood at the time when you experience it—for example, outrage—and afterward feel what sensation emerges inside your body that is related to that feeling—for instance your jaw is tight and shoulders are raised and tense. Doing as such encourages you to clear your head where you risk being cleared away by musings and instead tune in to your body where your instinct dwells.

Start rehearsing as an amateur onlooker, only seeing with intrigue what is befalling your body reactions various improvements and feelings. Guided body examines reflections are particularly useful in honing this ability. So are practices where you infer a particular memory and after that name and feel the feelings, it evokes inside your body. In these activities, consider your breathing, muscles, and pulse to perceive how your body responds and what that response lets you know. The information it holds is essential to contriving activity that is important and applicable to you.

Ask yourself, "What do I truly require here? What's significant for me?" This is one of those occasions when it has to be about you, so give yourself full consent to do as such. If you discover your focus moving to other individuals and their needs, notice and intentionally return your consideration back to being interested in what you need and want, since that is the place you will discover your instinct; focusing on these necessities serves to clear the pathway there effectively. To dispel any confusion concerning your intuition, it may be useful to initially experience the list of guilty parties above to distinguish the outside elements impacting you, recognizing them so you would then be able to set them aside for the occasion. Your instinct is a piece of your most astounding, smartest self, so ensure the attention is decisively on you.

The feeling of instinct resembles a sea tide and flow, exploring you toward a fulfilling life. When you find it, despite everything, you have to get in a boat and set sail to determine its full worth. After you answer the inquiry "What do I need now?" plan something to give yourself what you need. It may be the littlest advance, but size does not make a difference here. Small advances can really be helpful at first to slowly construct trust with your intuitive self which could be showing up for the first time just because of getting reacquainted with after an unfortunate relationship isolated you. What matters is that you are following your instinct.

Keep in mind that believing your instinct is a journey that will lead you back through these means frequently as conditions change and life keeps on moving. Think about your intuition as a muscle to fortify. With intentional practice and continuous use, it will turn out to be more dominant and better playing its role —managing your home to yourself.

Chapter 10: Self-Awareness

Before we begin discussing the origins of self-awareness, we should define what we're talking about. The kind of self-awareness we're discussing here is defined as having a clear understanding of your personality, including both your strengths and weaknesses as well as your thoughts, beliefs, emotions, and motivations. Being acutely self-aware means, in short, you know yourself, and you understand your motivations. It often requires taking a "deep dive" into what has shaped you and how that interacts with your emotions and thoughts to guide your behavior. It also means checking in with yourself at any moment to understand how events are impacting your emotional state. And, self-awareness is the foundation for emotional intelligence as well as self-leadership and mature adulthood. But where does this come from, and how do we develop it?

The Origin of Self-Awareness

Understanding self-awareness means understanding a little bit about the brain. There are three basic systems in the brain: the neocortex, which is our conscious mind where most of our thoughts happen; the limbic system, which is the subconscious "heart-centered" area where our emotions arise; and the basal ganglia, which is the unconscious "gut-centered" area where our instincts are activated. All three areas are involved in cultivating self-awareness. The neocortex is our conscious mind that we can access at any time. The limbic system is our subconscious mind, where we store emotions, value judgments, and memories. Lastly, the basal ganglia uses the information it receives from our gut to generate an unconscious instinctual response. It does so without checking with the other two regions of the brain

(Cascio 2015; Strecher 2015). You can begin to see how all of these regions can affect our feelings and our experience at any moment in time.

As we go through life accumulating experiences, we react to those experiences using all three systems. We respond with our conscious neocortex-- that is, we think about and rationalize the experience--and we use the subconscious limbic system to generate and store emotions we have around the experience, and those emotions generate a gut feeling that goes through the basal ganglia to activate appropriate instinctual responses. So, for example, if you feel fear, you may be analyzing what to do, but your negative emotions are being recorded and stored, and your gut feeling is stimulating an instinctual fear response. Most of this is happening on a subconscious or unconscious level. To generate self-awareness, we want to consciously access all of these areas in order to fully understand what we think and feel, and how that guides our actions.

As with learning any new skill, cultivating self-awareness means passing through four stages (Jeffrey 2019):

1. Unconscious incompetence--this is where you don't know how bad you are at something until you try. You don't know you can't play the piano until you play a few chords.

2. Conscious incompetence--this is where you are now aware of the fact that you are not good at doing something. You now understand that you can't play the piano.

3. Conscious competence--this is where you make a committed effort to learn a new skill, and because of your dedication and practice, you have now reached a level where you are reasonably good at this skill. You can play the piano. But, to get to this stage, you have to be willing to work through

some uncomfortable feelings that arise as a result of your conscious incompetence.

4. Unconscious competence--this is the brass ring. This is where you can now perform the skill effortlessly. You can sit down at the piano without sheet music and play songs easily. This is the stage where the magic happens.

Most people will give up when those uncomfortable feelings arise — as with any skill, developing self-awareness means passing through these stages.

Why We Lack Self-Awareness

As with any skill, cultivating self-awareness demands practice and dedication. It's uncomfortable to feel incompetent, and so, most people will give up at that stage of the process. And, many people fail to develop self-awareness because, although they try, they target only the conscious neocortex rather than all three systems. A conscious connection to all three systems is a must if we are to truly understand the root of our thoughts, feelings, and actions. If we increase our sensitivity to our emotions and instincts, we can more thoroughly explore our thoughts, beliefs, and biases, and it is only then that we can truly understand our behavior. Another problem in developing true self-awareness is that most people think they're self-aware, but very few are. According to a multi-year study by The Eurich Group, a group of psychologists who provide executive coaching and leadership development programs for businesses, only 10 to 15 percent of people actually exhibit the characteristics of self-awareness; this despite the fact that some 85 to 90 percent of people think they are self-aware (Eurich 2018). Real self-awareness means being able to identify your values, your goals, your flaws, and your motivations, all with an understanding of how your past has influenced your behavior. It means acting consciously in every area of your life, exploring emotions as they arise, digging to get at the reasons for your triggers, and acting with intentionality to not only preserve but grow your self-awareness. It means understanding your place in the universe and the impact your actions have on yourself and others. Developing this takes a lot of work, and many people have too much fear of those uncomfortable emotions and instinctive reactions that will undoubtedly happen along the way. That's why we lack self-awareness, but if you've come to the realization that you're among the 85 - 90 percent of those who have not developed their self-awareness, what can you do to cultivate it?

Gaining Self-Awareness Through Others

While there are many things that other people cannot do for you as you develop your self-awareness, one thing that they can do is help you understand some of your own strengths and weaknesses through effective feedback. Effective feedback does not mean criticism, but rather it is honest and kind, specific, not general, descriptive, not critical; and focused on helping you build your strengths rather than highlight your weaknesses. Having a life coach or even a trusted friend who can give you this kind of feedback can help you understand areas of your behavior that you might not even realize are affecting your life. It is often easier to see shortcomings in other people than it is to see them in yourself. This isn't necessarily because you're critical of other people, but because you can see the ways in which your good friends are limiting themselves or even sabotaging their own success, whereas they are too close to the situation. Likewise, you can be too close to your situation to understand how others see you. That's how others can help us to see things we might not be willing to look at without their help. Life coaches are people who are trained to help you with this kind of thing, but if you don't have one of those, you can ask a good friend to provide you with some effective feedback. You might try asking them to answer the following questions honestly:

1. What behaviors do you believe are limiting my potential?

2. How do you feel when you're talking to me?

3. What do you think I'm good at? What are some of my weaknesses?

4. If you had to describe me to someone, what would you say?

5. Is there anything you avoid saying to me because you're afraid of how I'll react?

These questions will prompt them to give you the kind of feedback you can use to see better the areas in your own life where you might want to make improvements. That can help as you move on to the next steps of mindfulness and daily self-reflection.

Creating a Daily Habit of Self-Reflection

One of the first things you need to be able to do in order to practice self-reflection is to learn how to find your center. You have to be able to quiet your mind and free yourself from distractions in order to be able to truly explore the roots or your behaviors, emotions, and thoughts. When you are centered, there is no tension, you're alert but calm, and you're in the present moment. To be able to achieve this, it's important to have a place to sit that is quiet and free from distractions. It's helpful to close your eyes, so you are not visually distracted, and to focus on your breathing. Most people have trouble with this part because it's difficult to keep your mind quiet. Your "monkey mind" starts chattering incessantly, jumping from thought to thought, just like the monkeys in the trees. The key to quieting the "monkey mind" lies not in judging yourself when those thoughts intrude, but rather in accepting them, noticing what they are, and letting them go. For example, as you start to quiet your mind, you might start thinking, "I've got to get that report done at work tomorrow." What should you do? As soon as you notice you've been distracted by a thought, just think to yourself, "Oh, that's planning--I'm planning right now what I've got to do tomorrow," and let it go-- visualize it actually rising up into the distance like smoke. Then, come back to your breath. Notice how fast you're breathing, how deep or shallow your breath is, and feel it coming in through the nose, traveling to the lungs, and coming back out again. Feel the rise and fall of your chest and your belly--that's right, breath into your belly. The goal is to achieve an even, rhythmic, deep breathing pattern.

Once you've got your breath flowing as you want, put your awareness on your body. Get in touch with the observer inside of yourself. Who is it that is noticing your thoughts? Who is it that notices your emotions? Use the observer to feel the surface you're sitting on, feel the contact with every part of your body. Don't just notice the contact with your backside, but your legs, your feet, the backs of your lower legs, your back against the back of the chair, and your hands resting on your legs. What do your legs and pants feel like? What does the fabric of the chair feel like on your legs? Can you feel your feet inside your shoes or socks? What do you hear? Try to divide the sounds you're hearing; try to hear those sounds we often relegate to background noise. Can you tease the different sounds apart? What are they? Do you find some of them to be annoying? What kind of reaction do they provoke in your body? Get in touch with the sensations in your body. Is there any area of pain, and what does that pain feel like? Is it sharp or dull? Is it constant or intermittent? Does it change? Try to notice these sensations before reacting to anything. For example, if you feel a sneeze coming on, try to notice what that feels like before you give in to the actual sneeze itself. Does your nose tickle? Do you feel a sharp inhale? Do your eyebrows rise as your eyes close? Notice what happens in your body before reacting to it. Feel the moment, and notice the stillness. Let yourself be still in the silence, and feel your body relax. Now, let the observer inform you about yourself.

What are you feeling? Is there something your mind just can't let go of? Navigate through as many emotions as arise in this state of mindfulness. Don't judge; just use the observer to notice what comes up and how what comes up feels in your body. For example, "Oh, that is shame.

I'm feeling ashamed. How does it feel? Where do I feel that in my body? I feel pain in my stomach, in my bowels, and pressure across my chest. I feel like I can't breathe fully. I feel like I have to breathe in little gulps of air. My face feels flushed, hot. Why am I feeling that shame? Oh, I remember, my parents always told me that was bad. I did that once when I was young, and they told me how disappointed they were in me. And I have never let that go. I've never forgiven myself or gotten over that. That's why I reacted the way I did today when my child did that. Now, I understand." This is how the observer can help you get at the deeper foundations behind your beliefs, emotions, and behaviors. This is what lies beneath your conscious thoughts; what comes from the limbic system and the basal ganglia. This is the kind of self-reflection you have to practice in order to cultivate true self-awareness. It can be difficult work, and it is at times, exhausting, but if you practice it daily, it will open you to a deeper understanding, compassion, and acceptance of yourself. And it will be worth it. You'll develop much deeper compassion for yourself and others, and you'll improve the relationship you have with yourself. You don't have to treat every emotion this way, but you'll know the ones that need your attention because they will create a strong physical reaction. You will feel that stomachache or the pressure across your chest. Those are signals that this is coming from a deeper place, a kind of core truth you've accepted about yourself. They'll also likely generate strong reactions. If you find yourself suddenly yelling at your partner, your child, or your coworker, that's a good indication you've been triggered. Likewise, if you find yourself yelling at yourself, something's up, and it's time to reflect on that.

This kind of mindfulness meditation should be practiced daily. It doesn't have to be for long, maybe only 15 minutes, but it is important to do this regularly. Just like with the affirmations, repetition is key. Another practice that is helpful is to keep a journal of your insights. Allow yourself to write anything you want. There are no judgments in this journal. Let your thoughts and insights flow. Sometimes you write something, and you don't realize the full impact of what you've written until you go back and read it the next day. And, you'll start to see your growth as your self-awareness skills develop. Practicing this mindfulness meditation and journaling will help you to really understand your life story and how the events that happened left their marks. These practices will also help you to develop new goals for your life. Mindfully meditating, practicing self-reflection, and documenting your insights and goals will help you improve at planning and prioritizing your needs. And, you'll gain more insight into the story of you, and just how you roll! This can then help you understand the things about yourself you'd like to change. That is the gift of self-awareness.

Chapter Summary

In this chapter, we've discussed self-awareness. We've defined it and discussed how to develop it. We've looked at the helpful practices of asking others to inform us about how they see us, and how to use mindfulness meditation and self-reflection to gain a deeper understanding of our thoughts, emotions, and behaviors.

We noted that the three areas of the brain involved in our behaviors and thoughts are the neocortex, where our conscious mind forms our thoughts, the limbic system, where our subconscious mind forms and stores our emotions and memories, and the basal ganglia, where our unconscious mind uses our gut feelings to stimulate instinctive physical reactions to our emotions. We've discussed that the path the self-awareness means we must form a more conscious connection with all three of these areas.

The next chapter will present more powerful, positive affirmations that you can use in your practice of mindfulness meditation and self-reflection.

Chapter 11: Self-Respect

Self-respect is a whole new different thing from respect. To put it plainly, self-respect is more of an internal thing. It is hardly noticeable from the outside, but the resulting action is noticeable. This is something you do for yourself; then it automatically radiates to others. Self-respect is a derivation of respect from the dictionary, but technically it is the other way round. Getting to know the fundamental components of respect helps in the application of self, including what respect itself entails.

Respect

The original definition of the word respect is to 'consider' or 'regard.' This word has since expanded in meaning to include definitions such as, 'to treat with deference,' 'to regard with esteem and dignity' or 'to fear.' The latter is used in a different context like religion or concerning authorities. Respect generally has two components, a subject and an object. These two can be used interchangeably, depending on what side we are viewing from. The subject responds to the object with or without respect, and the object shows a reaction. This kind of response by the subject is the way they feel or react in the presence of the object and towards the things the object does. Respect is of many dimensions, including beliefs, judgments, acknowledgments, emotions, feelings, motivations, dispositions and attitudes.

Several ways determine the amount of respect, if any, that is accorded the object. This should be a guideline for you as you cultivate self-respect. You are both the object and subject of yourself.

· **Appearance-** this is a form of cognitive respect where the subject weighs their surroundings, including the physical attributes of the object. It is then that the subject decides how to act and react to those features and generally towards the object.

· **Appraisal-** the subject weighs the object's level of deservingness. This is influenced by things like the title and age of the subject. Ordinarily, the subject would not accord the object this kind of respect if it were not for their status. This makes this kind of respect superficial; it is not genuine, but the object might not notice it for as long as the status quo remains.

· **Position-** this kind of respect is different from an appraisal in that the object is respected indirectly. In institutions, for example, those holding higher positions are respected by obeying the rules of that institution. This kind of respect does not normally go beyond the institution. Take a case where a husband and wife work in the same firm. The wife is the manager, while the husband is a low-ranking employee. The wife will be accorded unique respect at work, but that might not be reflected when the two go home in the evening. The respect doesn't end entirely, but it will take another dimension.

· **Demanded respect**- the subject is obliged to show the object respect irrespective. This is mostly shown in a military setting where junior officers must show respect to their seniors by following direct and indirect orders. This can also be regarded as indirect respect since the object merely follows rules set; it is more of respect for rules or orders and not the one that has come up with them.

· **Respect for barriers**- this is respect that is accorded to objects which the subject considers as obstacles. The subject merely shows respect to overcome these barriers as they might get hurt if they don't. A good example is when you are driving a jeep through a park, and you come across a pack of lions resting in the middle of the road. You either drive slowly past the fierce animals or risk being torn to pieces.

· **Respect for the character**- this is the most sincere and deserved form of respect. It is purely about how the subject carries themselves in the presence of the subject. The subject takes their time to evaluate the object's character before deciding on the amount of respect to give. However, as much as this kind of respect is sincere; it can be faked by the object especially if they want to meet certain objectives.

· Core Respect

· This is respect to the natural and inborn traits of yourself. It goes beyond only doing the right thing. It is a conviction to inculcate a morally acceptable code of behavior at all times. It also involves remaining firm and holding onto your fundamental principles at all times. Some of these principles are universal to the average people of character. Core respect is ingrained in them. They include:

· **Integrity-** this is the ability to stand up to your own beliefs and convictions by following your conscience and refusing to be bowed. It also involves remaining upright and courageous. A person of integrity sticks by their principles no matter what people say. They guard their reputation; however, costly it might seem. They don't do something wrong to please other people nor try to get what they want at the expense of others. It is the most effective tool in cultivating self-respect.

· **Courtesy-** people will always do to you what you do to them. Being courteous means being polite and practice good manners around people. No one respects a person that treats others with prejudice by insulting, ridiculing, and embarrassing them. A courteous person is someone that respects themselves.

· **Tolerance-** this involves accepting people for who they are without judging them based on gender, abilities, beliefs, and color. It also involves being ready to listen to other people's points of view the same way you'd want them to listen to yours. A person that lacks core respect will use the slightest opportunity they get to judge and discriminate against others.

· **Loyalty-** This is the ability and readiness to always stand up for people you love or associate with, such as friends, colleagues, and relatives. Being available to protect them and guard their interests whenever they are threatened. A loyal person will keep the secrets of the people close to them. They never betray people close to them nor let them do wrong things that might harm them. They don't backbite or act selfishly in front of their friends.

· **Honesty-** core respect involves being able to tell the truth even if it will turn against you. Being deceptive, lying, stealing, or cheating does more harm to you than the consequences of telling the truth. People will regard you highly if you are forthright and sincere at all times. It tells them that you value your dignity more than anything else.

· **Diplomacy-** being diplomatic is the ability to resolve conflicts amicably and fairly. Being diplomatic means, you can solve issues without the use of violence, and without being biased. It is a trait which only the strongest of character possesses. Someone that lacks core respect will let their anger get ahead of them whenever they are faced with disagreements. They will use force and threats to have their way. This will only paint a bad picture of their core respect, and they won't be respected either.

· **Reliability-** The ability to keep your word is a major booster of core respect. It means you are dependable and trustworthy. The opposite is someone that constantly goes back on their word, someone that does not honor their pledges and commitments. Such a person is a turn-off, and it points to a lack of core respect.

Personal Rules
These are the Dos and DON'Ts that guide your day to day life. You carry them everywhere you go. Coming up with your own rules and following them are two different things. It is more difficult to stick by the rules you have made compared to those made by someone else. It needs a lot of determination and discipline to follow your own rules. Unfortunately, you won't be able to live an exceptional life without these rules. Being able to follow the rules you have made means your level of self-respect is above per. Some of these rules are highlighted below.

· Plan your day before you start doing anything. This gives you a chance to balance things and accomplish all tasks for the day. It also ensures you don't get to waste time and end up engaging in negativity instead of doing meaningful things. The best way to plan your day is to come up with a timetable that covers the entire twenty-four hours. Make sure everything is allocated enough time.

· Prepare a stable sleeping schedule. Don't be the person to hop in and out of bed whenever you want. Always go to bed and wake up at the same time every day. This does not only help you develop a regular sleeping pattern, but it also supports the schedule you have come up with while planning your day. If you follow this rule, it means that you won't be skipping or overdoing tasks. However, as you come up with this sleeping schedule, make sure to provide enough time for sleep, this is roughly eight hours a day.

· Always have time for yourself every day. Remember that you are the most important component of these rules; it is all about you. Your physical self needs to be taken care of in the form of body exercises and monitoring. Your mental self needs care in the form of meditation to clear stress and anxiety. Your emotional self also needs to be looked into through soul-searching and monitoring your feelings. Set time for these little activities every day without fail, these activities can barely take an hour of your time. During this time, shut out all distractions like social media completely until you are done.

· Try and appreciate at least one person before the day ends. Show gratitude to people that have done even the slightest of the things for you that day. A simple smile and a 'thank you' is enough whenever someone shows you an act of kindness. If you are a religious person, show gratitude to your creator for the gift of life every morning before you get out of bed and immediately before you go to bed. Make this an everyday habit, and you will notice the kind of fulfilling the life you will be leading.

· Make your bed every time you wake up. Start your charity right from your bedroom. It is a simple act that carries a lot of weight concerning your day's plans. Spreading your bed neatly is the very first indication that you are ready to face the day in an organized manner.

Concordance
This is the urge to pursue your own goals and objectives not because someone is asking you to but because you believe they align with your underlying interests. It is a form of self-drive that is fundamental in inculcating self-respect. A self-concordant individual shows higher levels of subjective well-being. On the other hand, people that lack self-concordance are less effective in executing roles, be it for themselves or in places of work. Concordance leads to satisfaction since a self-concordant person will always come with own methods and techniques of meeting their objectives. This method is effective because it is well understood by the individual, unlike established methods that tend to be rigid.

This form of satisfaction is a result of respect for your interests and goals. The self-respecting person feels obliged to pursue those goals to the end without coercion. This yields surprisingly phenomenal results for the individual.

Boundaries

These are limits and rules that need to be watched to maintain a healthy relationship with yourself and others. There are those boundaries you draw that must not be crossed by others, and there are those that others have drawn, and you must not cross them. Boundaries are more like warnings and such come with consequences when crossed. This means that boundaries guard the interests of both parties, the party that draws them and the one that is meant not to cross. Boundaries are important because they guard our self-respect, ensures that we are kept away from harm, enables us to communicate our needs to other people, set limits in the relationship as well as ensure we make time for our time and space.

Boundary Boxes

Just like a Plassom Meter Boundary Box, the boundary boxes of self-respect are meant to protect you from outside threats. Having this box ensures you have a clean and conducive environment for self-growth and nourishment. The boundary is invisible physically, but it is also conspicuous in that you have made it known to the people around you. They are more of mental boundaries; they include the   following;

· **Personal beliefs and convictions-** set boundaries of the kind of thoughts you need to entertain. You won't know this boundary exists until it is crossed. Whenever you notice that your thoughts are wandering beyond who you are, more so to the negative, put a stop to them immediately. Stop the negative thing and divert your mind to something else that is positive.

· **Values**- your core values shape the character you become. Guard them jealously and refuse to be compromised whatsoever. Every value that is deemed positive is welcome, but put a stop to any that goes against who you are.

· **Opinions**- not every opinion needs to be entertained. If an idea undermines your self-respect, however pleasing it might sound, avoid it like the plague. Only allow those ideas that build your mind.

Boundary ranges

This is the extent to which your boundaries stretch. It involves setting the elastic limit for each boundary. If this limit is reached, then it means your self-respect is being threatened. It is okay to accommodate people, thoughts, and other objects but only up to a certain limit. You can, for example, allow someone to contributes their ideas towards a matter of mutual interest, but if you notice that their ideas are overriding yours, put a stop to that. A boundary has been crossed. It is

144

now   about   them   not   you.

Boundary levels
This is the level of relationship with yourself or others. It is the ability to only allow what you can accommodate. Learn to separate your feelings from those of other people to avoid being taken advantage of and losing your self-respect in the process. Letting your feelings be determined by other people's thoughts and feelings will only put you pressure to please them. Know when this boundary is being crossed and intervene appropriately.

Boundary circles
These are physical boundaries that are set to protect your personal space and body from the violation. Whenever these boundary circles are crossed, a person is left exposed to prejudice. In a way, this becomes your fault as those boundaries are not meant to be crossed. To guard your self-respect, always know who is supposed to touch you, how, and where they are supposed to touch you. Someone

that touches you against your will has crossed a boundary. Someone that touches you in the wrong place has crossed a boundary. Someone that touches you in a way that makes you feel uncomfortable has also crossed a boundary.

Your Remote Control
Achieving self-respect involves learning how to control various aspects of yourself with the touch of a button. Learn when to switch things on and off, depending on the effect they are having on your core being.

· Negative thoughts are not to be allowed in your mind for long. Go for that power off button immediately; you detect them. Then proceed to turn on positive and beautiful thoughts that will build you. You can alternate between different thoughts by simply switching channels. If an idea has become old and stale, switch to a new one that is relevant to your current situation.

· Your remote control allows you to regulate emotions. If a relationship is heading south, for example, reduce the feelings accorded to such a relationship by simply pressing the volume down button. This will save you a lot of agonies and guarantee self-respect when the relationship finally comes to an end. Similarly, turn up the feeling when you see a potential relationship.

· Regulate the volume when listening to people's opinions. Turn it off when you notice negativity and on when there is positivity.

Assertiveness

This is the ability to stand your ground while also respecting other people's opinions. Maintaining that balance does not only boost the level of respect accorded to you, but it also shows that you have a high level of self-respect. Assertiveness gives a win-win situation where both parties come out with their pride intact. This makes it an effective way guarding one's self-respect. You can practice assertiveness by following these rules;

· Always know what you want before the negotiation process starts. This involves being familiar with your rights and underlying interests. Let the other party know these needs and notice their reaction. Make sure you confidently voice this to drive the point home.

· Learn to say NOWHERE it is necessary and explain why you are taking that stand, be positive in your explanation.

· Be open to criticism the same way you are open to compliments.

· Try to know what the other party's interests are. This might not be easy to know, but you can ask and allow them to state their case without judgment and interruption.

· Weigh both sides and try not to be biased. Leaning on either side will undermine your self-respect. Even if you win as a result of being biased, you'd have lost the respect of the other party and respect for yourself.

Testing Boundaries

The strength of the boundaries you set can only be determined by carrying out a random test on them. This should be done in a controlled manner to avoid escalating things beyond control. Testing boundaries allows you to identify and seal loopholes. It also helps you come up with appropriate measures to respond when those boundaries are crossed.

Skills to Build Better Boundaries
Building boundaries requires effective skills to avoid having them broken easily. Some of these skills include:

· Know where you begin and end. This allows you to monitor your boundaries with ease.

· Separate your identity from other people. It gives you a chance to know what is good for you and what is not. It also protects you from unhealthy competition.

· Understand that you are entirely responsible for yourself. The strength of the boundaries determines the level of safety you get.

· Overcome feelings of guilt, embarrassment, and selfishness before drawing a boundary. This clears your mind and enables you to become firm when guarding those boundaries.

· Support and reward those people that respect your boundaries and rebuke those that do not respect them. This allows you to only associate with people that value and respect you.

Healthy Relationship

This is a relationship where your rights and interests are respected. It is a relationship where the right to set boundaries is not judged as selfish. A healthy relationship helps you cultivate self-respect because the other party respects your character and gives you credit for it, they will then reciprocate in kind. Lack of self-respect, on the other hand, will only expose you to toxic relationships where no one respects you. These are the tips for are a healthy relationship.

· Learn to listen to the other person the same way you want them to listen to you.

· Do not be quick to judge. Put yourself in their shoes first before concluding.

· Accept your flaws and welcome criticism.

· Do not put your interests first at the expense of the other person's. Create some balance to avoid appearing selfish and greedy.

· Respect people's boundaries if you want yours to be respected.

Improving My Support System

Your support system is the people and objects that help you build self-respect by respecting you. They understand your right to set boundaries, and they respect those boundaries. You can support them by respecting their boundaries, as well. Another way of improving your support system is by showing appreciation to those that support you. This can be in the form of small gifts and complementary statements. Sometimes a simple 'thank you' will work just fine.

Forgiveness

To earn more respect from people around you, learn to pardon them whenever they wrong you. Softening your heart drives some form of guilt through them, and they might not end up repeating the same mistake. It also makes them say 'sorry' when they make mistakes in the future. They know you will forgive them. This might be viewed as encouraging repeating of mistakes, but look at it from this angle, someone makes a mistake and act as if nothing has happened. It will prick you.

Apologize

Apologizing for making a mistake or wronging someone does not make you weak. It means you are strong enough to realize that you are an ordinary human that is prone to errors. It means you respect the feelings of others by acknowledging that you might have hurt their feelings as a result of that mistake. They will respect you for this and might feel obliged to forgive you in the future. However, the act of apologizing does more to you as a person than those you are apologizing to. It shows that you respect yourself just like you respect others. Apologizing releases you from the clasp of guilt and embarrassment that results from being insensitive to the feelings of others.

Chapter 12: How To Overcome Low Self Esteem

If you find out that you have low self-esteem, it influences each part of your life and detracts from your pleasure and bliss. Beating low self-esteem can be cultivated if someone is eager to work at it. It doesn't occur incidentally, and it takes a great deal of work and persistence, however, the result is well worth the exertion.

Improving Your Self-Esteem

1. Perceive that numerous people experience the ill effects of low self-esteem.

You are not the only one. In an ongoing report, research found that 4% of single ladies around the globe see themselves as beautiful.

2. Recognize the musings, sentiments, physical indications, and practices related to low self-esteem.

Numerous individuals mistake these musings, practices, and sentiments with characteristics. In any case, negative considerations are not equivalent to actual characteristics. These kinds of contemplations, sentiments, physical signs, and practices resemble 'indications' of low self-esteem.

Perceiving the side effects will enable you to recognize what musings, emotions, and practices should be focused on for development.

3. Tune in to your inward monologue.

At the point when a large number of the accompanying musings happen, it resembles you're hearing a voice inside your head. These considerations are frequently programmed, practically like a reflex.

- I'm excessively feeble/not gifted enough/not savvy enough.

- I trust they don't believe I'm an American.

- I'm excessively fat/meager/old/youthful/and so on.

- Everything is my shortcoming.

- I think I must be impeccable when I perform at my specific employment.

- My supervisor doesn't care for my report. I should be a complete disappointment at my specific employment.

- Why have a go at meeting new individuals? They won't care for me.

4. Pinpoint how it is you feel about yourself.

Emotions, similar to musings, regularly originate from an internal discourse that doesn't precisely mirror the facts.

- I feel so embarrassed that my manager didn't care for my report.

- I'm so irate at myself that my manager didn't care for my report.

- I'm so baffled at my manager censuring me.

- I feel restless/frozen when I'm with people who I don't know since they're most likely pondering how fat I am.

- I'm not sufficiently able to contend, so I won't attempt.

- I feel on edge more often than not.

5. Search for physical signs that identify with low self-esteem.
The next might be physical signs that you have low self-esteem.

- I can't rest more often than not.

- I am worn out more often than not.

- My body feels tense.

At the point when I meet a new individual (or I'm in another awkward circumstance):

- I sweat lavishly.

- The room turns.

- I can't regain some composure.

- I redden a great deal.

- I feel like my heart is going to explode from out of my chest.

6. Survey your conduct to check whether your self-esteem is impacting your life.

If you find that at least one of these conduct proclamations concern you, your self-esteem might be greatly affecting the way you live.

- I don't go out/I don't care for individuals to see me, or me them.

- I experience difficulty in deciding.

- I don't feel good communicating my suppositions or supporting myself.

- I don't believe I'm fit for taking care of a new position, regardless of whether it is an advancement.

- I get agitated without any problem.

- I contend with the individuals throughout my life a lot.

- I get protective and shout at my family.

- My companion calls me 'Feline' constantly and I don't care for it, yet I'm apprehensive of the fact that if I say anything, she won't be my companion.

- I'm too self-cognizant to engage in sexual relations.

- I engage in sexual relations in any event when I would prefer not to.

- All that I do must be great.

- I eat well past being full.

- I can't eat more than one supper daily or I'll get excessively fat.

7. Distinguish your negative musings.

Regardless of whether you understand it or not, your considerations in your mind are catching you inside the pattern of low self-esteem. To feel improved, it's good to recognize when these kinds of considerations are going on, and discover approaches to conquer them. There are some common negative self-articulations you can get comfortable with, so if you run over some of them, you can target them for elimination.

8. Try not to be a nagger, putter-killjoy, or a name-guest.

Envision you have a 'companion' who is continually close by, and this companion continually upbraids you. The person calls you awful names, reveals to you that you are doing everything incorrectly, you're good for nothing, you'll accomplish nothing, and you're unlikable. Wouldn't that get you down?

9. Abstain from being a generalist.

The generalist will make a mistake, an event where the person in question didn't perform to desires or exceed expectations. For instance, if an individual strides into a pothole, she may have these contemplations that she was summing up: "For what reason do things like this consistently transpire? I'm simply reviled. I never have any good karma whatsoever."

10. Battle the inclination to be a comparer.

People who contrast consistently feel insufficient because individuals of this kind of thought design are constantly contrasting themselves and others, and accepting that everybody around them is superior to them.

For example, a comparer may state this: "Take a look at that. My neighbor has a Hemi truck. I don't know if I would ever bear the cost of one of those. I'm such a disappointment."

11. Evade the voice that transforms you into a person that catastrophizes.

People who catastrophize make conclusions about their whole lives and depend on one episode.

This is what a catastrophizer may think: "I got a B in this class rather than an A. I'll never get a new line of work."

12. Recall that you are not a mind reader.

Psyche readers consistently believe that people think the most noticeably awful thing about them. In actuality, we don't generally have the foggiest idea of what others are thinking.

Mind readers tend to make suspicions about what others are thinking or the reasons they are getting things done, and the brain reader considerations are constantly slanted: "That person is gazing at me. He's most likely reasoning what a monstrosity I am."

13. Focus on wiping out negative musings.

With this negative information, it's no big surprise self-esteem endures. If you perceive your ineffective idea designs, you can battle them. It requires some investment and tolerance because changing old propensities takes a great deal of work. Making it in little strides is exceptionally useful.

It's simpler to do small amounts of progress, and it's simpler to start treating yourself well by intuition in a positive manner.

14. Separate among supposition and fact.

Ordinarily, it tends to be hard to perceive what is a feeling and what is a fact. Our inward considerations are frequently conclusions, regardless of whether we think they are facts.

A fact is an unquestionable explanation, for example, "I am twenty-two years of age." You have the birth declaration to demonstrate it.

Assessments are not unquestionable. A case of an assessment is: "I'm constantly inept."

This announcement is refutable. Some may believe it's not, and they will offer proof of times where they believe they were idiotic, for example, "I'm so inept, I tumbled off the phase when I was eight."

However, while investigating this experience, a person can get familiar with a couple of things, for example, an adult was answerable for supervising the task, so that person ought to have thought about your well-being.

People are not great and commit errors. Indeed, even Einstein has conceded a few mistakes in his career. This shows nobody is extremely dumb if they commit errors. Indeed, even virtuoso's commit errors.

Regardless of whether you have encounters supporting your negative convictions, you ought to also have encounters supporting when you've settled on incredible decisions and have done some extremely shrewd things.

Utilizing a Journal to Improve Self-Esteem
1. Start a self-esteem journal.

Since you know a few reasons why the loss of self-esteem happens and the fundamental negative considerations that are answerable for sustaining low self-esteem, you can start the procedure to change your convictions about yourself. This procedure may be simpler to do on the PC, so you can change the association around so it sounds good to you without beginning your journal once more. A spreadsheet position is a decent method to keep your musings organized and permits you a lot of space to experiment.

2. Become a negative idea investigator.

For a couple of days, monitor your negative musings. You can keep these in a paper scratchpad, on a calendar function on a PC or your iPad. Watch all the negative articulations you make to yourself. In a situation where you don't remember them by type, it's alright. Record the announcement at any rate.

For instance, one of the things on the rundown was, "I'm going to come up short if I want to or even attempt to make it as an essayist," with related contemplations: "Why is this even trouble? Nobody will like it in any case. Nobody has anything unique to state in any case. It's been composed before."

3. Arrange your list.

Title this section: 'Negative Thoughts'. Put the contemplations into request, the highest point of the page containing the ones that trouble you the most, and the base musings that make you the least resentful. If you see various kinds of articulations that share something for all intents and purpose, bunch them together.

For instance, "I will fall flat if I attempt to make it as an author" is at the highest priority on the list. All related negative considerations can be incorporated with this idea, yet the lead sentence can be thought of as the title for this estimation.

4. Discover the foundation of each negative idea.

Make a section close to your 'Negative Thoughts' segment and call it 'Memory/Experience Associated With This Thought'. A person or experience may ring a bell. Record it. If not, simply leave it clear. Understanding where you've been will assist you with acknowledging why you feel the way you do.

For instance, "My dad disclosed to me I would come up short if I end up attempting to be an author."

Keep in mind, if you recall that somebody expressed a negative remark to you, this isn't a fact! It's just their assessment, and you will have the option to figure out how to disprove it.

Note: If this progression makes you so annoyed that it's hard for you to work on for the remainder of the day or week, or makes it hard for you to proceed, stop and look for proficient treatment.

5. Distinguish emotions related to each idea.

In the following section, titled 'The Way This Thought Makes Me Feel', record any emotions you may have related to this negative proclamation. This will assist you with the understanding that your contemplations influence your emotions.

For instance, "It makes me want to surrender."

6. Distinguish your practices.

The following section state, 'How I Act When I Think and Feel Like This'. Then attempt to think about an ongoing occasion that will assist you in acknowledging how you act. Do you get tranquil? Do you shout? Do you cry? Do you stay away from eye to eye connection with individuals? This will assist you with perceiving how your considerations and emotions are interconnected with the way with which you act.

For instance, "When I saw challenges or solicitations to compose, I disregarded them even though I need to be an author more than anything else."

7. Alter your reasoning.

It's an ideal opportunity to counter your negative suppositions and encounters with positive ones, which will assist you with understanding that the negative explanations are conclusions that hold you down and that you should quit trusting in these negative assessments you have framed yourself with.

8. Counter the pessimism.

Add a section to your journal called 'Rude awakening'. In this segment, put down any characteristic, great memory, achievement, or whatever else that is positive to counteract your negative conviction. If you locate a counter to your conviction, at that point your negative conviction won't hold any fact or legitimacy in your life. The idea you accepted to be a flat-out principle is not the standard.

For instance, "I have had five sonnets distributed, universally! Ha! Take that! I have also had four magazine articles distributed. It's false all things considered. I won't come up short. I've just succeeded!"

9. Make a positive action plan.

In your last section, you can put what you know enthusiastically with 'What I Will Do Now'. For this segment, be liberal with your thoughts on what you will do starting now and into the foreseeable future.

For instance, "I will do all that I can to ensure I succeed. I will return to class for my master's certificate. I will investigate where I can compose and get my articles distributed, and I won't surrender until I get paid work. I will search for composing work. I will participate in challenges. I won't surrender until I win one."

10. Concentrate on your positive traits.

Give a segment of your journal (or another tab in your spreadsheet) to composing positive things about yourself. Rewrite or make a rundown of your positive characteristics. Anything that will cause you to feel great about yourself and assist you with acknowledging what your identity is, the thing that you've achieved, and how far you've come in your life can be composed on this page. You may decide to concentrate on a few or the entirety of the accompanying:

- Your accomplishments. (for the afternoon, week, month, year.)

- I spared my organization 7,000,000 dollars this year.

- I invested energy with my children consistently.

- I figured out how to deal with my stress so I feel great most days.

- I won an honor.

- I grinned at another person I didn't know today, even though this is hard for me.

- Your properties and qualities.

- I have a bubbly character.

- I can offer an extraordinary compliment.

- I am a great listener.

- I know how to cause the ones I love to feel good.

11. Distinguish areas that you might want to improve.

It is imperative to address ways that you might want to improve without excessively concentrating on thoughts of solidarity or shortcoming. Accepting we are frail or insufficient in one way or another will be another self-esteem trap. It's awful that this self-vanquishing thought is upheld all through our general public.

Quit considering yourself as far as shortcomings and rather consider territories you might want to improve, and simply because transforming them will fulfill you.

Making objectives for change isn't tied in with fixing something that is broken. It's tied in with doing things that will assist you with working more effectively in your life and assist you with having solid connections, which helps your self-esteem and joy.

In your journal, either make another tab in your spreadsheet—or another page in your paper journal—and consider it the title of this segment: 'Zones I Would Like to Improve'. Then compose underneath it: 'Although it will satisfy me'.

A few instances of progress objectives that are not excessively centered around shortcomings are: I might want to...

- Oversee stress all the more effectively.

- Work on sorting out my desk work.

- Work on getting more organized.

- Make sure to accomplish something I truly appreciate once per day and not feel regretful about it.

- Improve my child-bearing aptitudes.

Changing Your Relationships
1. Surround yourself with positive people.

If you have contrary contemplations in your mind, it's conceivable you have people around you who are expressing similar sorts of negative messages about you, even dear loved ones. As you're improving your self-esteem, if it's conceivable, limit contact with individuals you notice are stating negative comments to you, regardless of whether they are near you or are busy working.

2. Consider negative articulations from others as a ten-pound load.

In a situation where you put on a ten-pound weight for each antagonistic explanation, and you are encircled by people who put you down. In the long run, it turns out to be harder to lift yourself.

Expelling yourself from the weight of tuning in and identifying with antagonistic individuals will cause you to feel lighter since you don't need to hold up under the heaviness of their negative remarks, their negative decisions towards you, or their reluctance to approach you with deference.

Assertiveness urges others to approach you with deference, which will help support positive self-esteem. To put it plainly, assertiveness prevents people's other awful practices from affecting you just as it causes you have sound correspondences with the people around you. You can use a couple of various procedures to practice assertive indifference.

3. Utilize 'I' rather than 'you'.

Instead of saying, "You didn't take out the waste the previous evening," you can state, "I feel upset when guarantees are made and aren't seen through."

The primary proclamation can be taken as an assault and increment the audience's defensiveness. The second is sharing your emotions, and telling the individual what the person in question did to add to those sentiments.

4. Tune in and be eager to settle.

Consider how the people you talk with feel and be eager to reach an accord that satisfies both of you.

For example, if your companion requests that you drive him to the store, you can say, "I can't at present; I have a class. I can drive you a short time later. Would that be alright?"

5. Be tireless without getting aggressive.

You can say no, and you can go for your privileges without hollering, and without surrendering. In case you're experiencing difficulty expressing what is on your mind, *Psychology Tools* suggests utilizing a 'broken record' approach, where you keep up consideration and a wonderful tone.

For instance, if your nearby market sold you an awful bit of meat and won't acknowledge its return, you can say, "I understand. I would like a discount." If after a few endeavors you don't see your outcomes, you can attempt an announcement like this, "If you would prefer not to give me a discount, that is your decision. I can decide to call the Health Department, however, I'd prefer not to. Which would be simpler for the two of us?"

6. Set individual boundaries.

It's your obligation to let your loved ones—as well as associates, friends, and collaborators—how you need to be dealt with. A few practices from others can directly affect your self-esteem if you hear it long enough.

For example, if you conclude you don't need others calling you names, you can tell them you don't care for it and you will make a move or take action if they do not desist from their current path.

If this type of obnoxious attack doesn't stop, make a move, and tell somebody with power that can support you. In case you're grinding away, record a provocation objection. In case you're an understudy, tell your parents, an educator, or your head. Maybe it's a companion, but your companion probably wouldn't have understood that their actions were getting you upset. It's constantly justified despite all the trouble to tell individuals how you feel.

Improving Your Lifestyle

1. Set aside a few minutes for yourself, regardless of whether you are a parent.

Numerous guardians mistakenly remove themselves from the condition when thinking about their children. It's normal to need to concentrate to give them the most ideal condition. Be that as it may, if you quit concentrating and disregard yourself, this can detract you from being the parent you truly need to be.

Guardians are educators to their children. With the goal for instructors to be genuinely powerful, educators must have a type of skill. Also, your very own propensities may come off on them, and this incorporates the awful ones just as the great ones.

Deciding to deal with yourself a couple of moments daily is everything necessary and not exclusively to raise your self-esteem, yet in addition to fill in as an extraordinary model for your children.

If you don't have children, dealing with yourself will assist you with feeling much improved and merits the exertion.

2. Pick healthy nourishments.

Eating healthy nourishment choices may take some underlying arranging from the start that you intend to do a whole way of life makeover. In any case, this can be overwhelming for effectively occupied, stressed-out individuals.

Rather than keeping convoluted arrangements of things you eat or things you ought to eat, settle on a decision to pick a healthy choice at each dinner and bite.

Evade nourishments like confections, pop, cake, doughnuts, and baked goods, which lead to huge vitality crashes, potential cerebral pains, and offer no sustenance, conceivable ailment, and included calories.

3. Eat more natural products, veggies, lean meats, and vegetables.

Consider them throughout the day. Vitality and bottomless sustenance for your body will empower you to stay aware of your activity and children, and ensure your body against sicknesses. This will expand your life so you can appreciate more time with your family.

4. Take a stab at a reasonable eating routine.

A decent meal will give you the nourishment needs to keep you healthier and more joyful. Here is a general rule for what you ought to endeavor to eat:

- 1 serving of organic product or veggies at each supper. Veggies and organic products also offer a touch of protein, starches, and plant-sourced fiber.

- 1 serving of lean protein at each feast. (vegetables, lean meats, low-fat dairy.) Vegetables and low-fat dairy offers a few sugars.

- 2 servings of starches for every day. (yams and entire oats are less handled and superior to entire wheat.)

- A touch of healthy fats like olive and canola oils, avocados, nuts. Nuts give a few starches just as healthy fats.

5. Consider your nourishment decisions.
At each supper, stop yourself, and inquire as to why you need to place unhealthy nourishments in your body.
A few purposes behind wandering from a healthy eating routine are:

- Healthy nourishment decisions are not accessible at gas stops.

- I'm eager now and I don't have the opportunity to run out/make a healthy supper.

A touch of arranging at the supermarket could help keep this from happening:

- Purchase hacked veggies like cleaved lettuce and infant carrots for a brisk serving of mixed greens.

- Purchase nuts or sunflower seeds for a fast fiber/protein/healthy fats help. You can add them to your plate of mixed greens for an additional crunch.

- Numerous natural products are versatile like bananas and apples.

6. Fight off sweet desires.
This can appear to be an unfavorable undertaking to certain individuals. In addition to the fact that we become connected to nourishments since it gives us comfort (like mother's chocolate chip treats), once your body is in an unhealthy cycle, handled nourishments like white

sugar play hormonal ruin on your body and the wanting for desserts cycle becomes self-sustaining. When you're battling your body to end the sweet yearnings, this can cause us to feel like we're not in charge of what we eat, which can bring down self-esteem. If for some reason, you have desires for something sugar-loaded, here are a few hints to wean yourself off of that white sugar:

Need something sweet toward the beginning of the day? Supplant your cake, sugar-loaded grain, and espresso cake with oats beat with Stevia, cinnamon, natural product, and milk. If you don't care for oats (a few people don't care for the mush factor), attempt earthy colored rice.

Need an evening shot of sugar? Attempt a few dates and nuts.

Need an after-supper dessert? Attempt two or three squares of dull chocolate (pick the brand with minimal measure of sugar) and nutty spread. Need to include somewhat more pleasantness? Liquefy your chocolate, mix in the nutty spread, and include some agave nectar or Stevia.

Not sweet enough? You can also blend in certain raisins to expand the yum factor even more, but when necessary.

7. Get your body going.

Setting aside some effort to go to the rec center may appear to be infeasible for caught up with working mothers and fathers. That is alright. You don't need to go to the exercise center to be fit as a fiddle. It's important to have more vitality, feel better, battle sickness, and have the option to stay aware of the requests of your bustling life. There are even schedules accessible that are ten minutes or less. You can do these schedules each day since they won't exhaust the body. Here are a couple of instances of fast yet successful exercise programs:

Daily Workouts Fitness Trainer Free: This is a downloadable application accessible on apple   store. https://apps.apple.com/us/app/daily-workouts-fitness-trainer/id469068059
Chatelaine Ten Minute Fitness: This downloadable application from iTunes is a global   smash   hit.

https://itunes.apple.com/ca/app/chatelaine-10-minute-fitness/id643853756?mt=8
The 7 Min Workout: This site reveals to you which basic activities to do and times your whole seven-minute meeting for you. It's so quick, you don't have the opportunity to illuminate the word minute. Also, it offers the 7 Min diet if you offer your first name and email address.
http://www.7-min.com/
Caution: These exercises are short, however, they can be thorough. Along these lines, it's ideal to check with your PCP if you have a condition you are being treated for, or whether you are over forty.

8. Remain well-prepped.

It may sound odd, however, brushing your teeth, washing up, styling your hair, wearing attire that is open to giving yourself a nail treatment, and dealing with your body all in all lifts your self-esteem.

If you truly feel better and put forth attempts to keep up your appearance, realizing you smell extraordinary in your preferred fragrance or cologne, or that your hair is delicate and touchable, or your eyes look more green since you're wearing your preferred green shirt can give you a lift for the afternoon.

Finding Appropriate Therapy

1. Go to treatment to support your self-esteem.

If you are experiencing difficulty with raising your self-esteem or want to see faster improvement, think about going to a proficient treatment. Successful treatment has appeared to have a huge impact on raising self-esteem.

You may also need to find support in keeping your journal, so you understand that there are subjects that you can't confront, or in the likelihood that you are attempting to confront them, they set you back enough to cause a disturbance in your life as you delve back on them.

Also, if you have a psychological issue like melancholy, anxiety, or different sorts of disarranges, this can affect your self-esteem. Getting treatment for a psychological issue can improve in an amazing nature.

2. Attempt Cognitive Behavioral Therapy.

Cognitive behavioral therapy (CBT) has been demonstrated to be powerful at developing self-esteem. CBT addresses programmed negative musings. These musings are the considerations that happen like a reflex when confronted with life circumstances.

For instance, if an individual with low self-esteem needs to prepare for a test in school, the individual may say, "I don't have a clue why I'm irritating. I'll get an F at any rate."

While experiencing CBT treatment, the therapist, who will be a guide or clinician, works in partnership with the customer to change those programmed beliefs. The advocate may propose testing the customer's theory—the customer will bomb regardless of how hard the customer examines. Help the customer with time management, stress abilities, and track progress until the understudy steps through the exam.

Different strategies utilized for CBT are unwinding methods (breathing activities), representation (mental practicing), and experiencing youth encounters to distinguish where the negative musings began. Recognizing the root of the negative contemplations forestalls self-esteem 'relapses'.

CBT is useful for people who don't have complex issues. Besides, CBT is useful for treating a few kinds of issues like discouragement and anxiety.

CBT may also be unreasonably organized for certain individuals.

3. Find psychodynamic treatment.

With psychodynamic therapy, treatment plans are custom-fitted to every individual and their individual needs. In a psychodynamic meeting, the customer is permitted to investigate all issues emerging for that day. The clinician enables the customer to search for conduct, thought, and emotional examples identified with that issue. Youth issues and occasions are frequently investigated to enable the customer to see how the past influences them and connects to their present.

For individuals who have complex issues or might want an individualized arrangement customized to their requirements, psychodynamic treatment may be better than CBT.

Psychodynamic treatment is a powerful method to use with an assortment of conditions and with patients with issues of changing unpredictability.

Distinguishing Low Self-Esteem

1. Know the potential impacts of low self-esteem.

Having low self-esteem doesn't simply impact your emotional state at some random second; it can have a long-running impact on your life. Understanding the potential impacts of low self-esteem may help inspire you to improve your viewpoint now. Low self-esteem may lead individuals to do any of the following:

- Endure injurious connections since they believe they are meriting the treatment or don't merit better treatment.

- Bully or misuse others.

- Being hesitant to take on objectives, destinations, or dreams since they don't think they can accomplish them.

- Become sticklers to compensate for their apparent blemishes.

- Continuously feel self-cognizant around others, be excessively distracted with their appearance, or imagine that others consider them.

- Continually search for markers that others don't care for them or ineffectively consider them.

- Think they are an act of futility.

- Have a low limit for stress.

Disregard their cleanliness or take part in activities that hurt their body, for example, drinking unnecessary liquor, smoking tobacco, or endeavoring self-destruction.

2. Pinpoint the base of your self-esteem issue.

Usually, low self-esteem begins with outer occasions. Individuals are not brought into the world with low self-esteem. It starts with our necessities not being met, negative feedback from others, or believing that a negative life occasion is our flaw.

For instance, children may reprimand themselves for their parent's separation or guardians feel powerless to enable their children to process their emotions.

Children who experience childhood in destitution and offspring of minorities are frequently at higher risk for growing low self-esteem.

3. Comprehend the low self-esteem cycle.

At the point when children (or adults) initially start to scrutinize their value, it is feasible for others or life occasions to fortify the negative sentiments, which can harden self-convictions that lead to low self-esteem.

4. Recollect how your parents treated you.

Guardians have been found to have the most grounded effect on people's self-esteem. Children's impressions of themselves are shaped with the assistance of their folks. There are a few unique sorts of parental practices that add to low self-esteem.

Frequently, when children are brought up in a severe home that doesn't give them emotional help, their self-esteem suffers. At the point when children and adults have emotional help, their emotional needs are met. Emotional help can be appeared from various perspectives, for example, saying, "I love you", or "I'm glad for you"; helping kids with their sentiments and emotions, and how to adapt, and simply being there for them.

Emotional requirements are genuine necessities individuals have as they develop, along with physical (nourishment and drink) and mental (learning, critical thinking, and training) needs. Focusing on emotional necessities, just as physical and mental needs, assists children with feeling acknowledged and regarded.

5. Perceive cases of disgrace in your life.

Shaming is a typical child-bearing apparatus to help control the conduct of children. For example, open disgracing of children via web-based networking media has become normal. Disgracing happens when somebody, for example, a guardian, parent, instructor, or other powerful figures, or different friends, causes you to feel like you are a horrendous individual for carrying on in a specific way or committing an error.

For instance, and if for some reason, you don't show up on time to your work, your manager may cause you to feel embarrassed if he says, "You are not a dependable individual", as opposed to, "You have to come into work before. Take a stab at showing up to work thirty minutes sooner. If anything turns out badly, you'll have that extra time."

While disgracing is socially acknowledged, it is an injurious conduct, and frequently happens with other harsh practices that produce the sentiment of being disgraced. For instance, creator Beverly Engel reviews her mom hitting her before her neighbors, or rebuffing her with open presentations of shouting when she committed an error. These rates delivered sentiments of disgrace.

6. Distinguish maltreatment in past connections.

Harsh relationship designs are regularly the reason for low self-esteem. Patterns like scolding, deprecating, controlling, shouting, or reprimanding would all be able to add to people's contemplations of themselves. After some time, when these practices are rehashed again and again, the casualty may accept this negative information.

Harsh connections can also influence adults. The connections we have in adulthood frequently mirror our youthful connections. Relationship designs are shaped in youth, which influences our desires for our future connections.

7. Recognize occasions of horrible showing from before.

At the point when people reliably perform inadequately at an errand, at school, or an occupation, this can prompt lost self-esteem. It has been found over many years of research examinations that an industrious, however moderate, interface between poor scholarly execution and low self-esteem.

This isn't unexpected, considering the school is part of the greater part of our lives and for a larger part of our childhoods during our early stages in life.

8. Comprehend the impact of life occasions on your self-esteem.

Life occasions—even ones that are outside one's ability to control—frequently impact self-esteem. Job misfortune, monetary troubles, a separation, physical and psychological maladjustment, constant torment, and handicaps are kinds of circumstances that can be incessantly stressful and erode at a person's self-esteem.

Separation, occasions that produce injury like being in a vehicle or work mishap, being the survivor of an assault, or the demise of a relative or companion, can influence self-esteem too.

Money related stress and living in a financially discouraged zone can also influence self-esteem.

9. Survey your encounters of social acknowledgment.

Social acknowledgment, or the measure of dismissal encounters, has been found to have consequences for self-esteem. This has been found when contrasting the jobless with the utilized, yet different impacts like having a social disgrace (liquor abuse, psychological maladjustment), have been found to influence self-esteem.

10. Realize that your assessment of your physical appearance is associated with your self-esteem.

Physical appearance can influence one's self-esteem. It has been uncovered through research that there is an acknowledged definition for magnificence. While these standards are socially impacted, there is a socially acknowledged thought for excellence.

If an individual gets a great deal of dismissal or acknowledgment for their appearance, this could have an impact on a person's self-worth.

Research has discovered that when people assess their physical appearance, it is reliably slanted towards the negative and may not definitively reflect our true qualities. So it goes without saying, most people are too critical of their physical looks.

11. Note situations of bullying in your past. Because of the persistent harassment, bullying adds to low self-esteem. There are repercussions to self-esteem for both the victim and the bully in this vicious cycle.

Recipients of bullying often have to live for years with the memories of them being bullied. They often feel humiliated about the abuse and assaults.

Most bullies also suffer from low self-esteem and feel more behind the wheel when they victimize others.

Lightning Source UK Ltd.
Milton Keynes UK
UKHW020636070422
401231UK00009B/483